L.I.F.E. Fit, The Process takes you through the famo

weight loss and body toning programme designed w

the tools you need to 'Lose It ForEver' A programme that works seamlessly into real family life, without the need for drastic food changes or complicated meal plans.

Instead of isolating you from the rest of your family through extreme food restrictions or calorie counting regimes, L.I.F.E. Fit creates an opportunity for you to introduce a healthy lifestyle for everyone at home, while you lose weight.

L.I.F.E. Fit understands that as a parent your weight loss journey is not just about you anymore and that everything you do has to incorporate and benefit your children too. There is no point undertaking a new healthy regime if your children do not benefit from it and this is where L.I.F.E. Fit differs from other weight loss programmes. It is designed to benefit the entire family. The L.I.F.E. Fit approach is built upon eating well, exercising right and being a great example to your children.

At last. A weight loss and fitness programme designed specifically for Mums! A programme that allows for child routines and busy family life. A programme that allows children to benefit from mum's healthy body transformation. A programme that brings health and fitness into the heart of the home while Mum loses the unwanted body fat. A weight loss programme designed to fit seamlessly into the day of a busy Mum taking into account family mealtimes, without flipping family routine upside down. A programme that works with real life and makes it a real healthier life, for the whole family. No more yo-yo dieting!

Above all, this is a programme that delivers real weight loss and body toning results that are completely sustainable, meaning your results are for the long-term! Mums, this is the last home fitness programme you will ever need to follow!

To all you real-life mums whose paths I have been fortunate enough to cross. Your relentless determination to take control of your daily life, your bodies and your family's health together with your everlasting enthusiasm and endless dedication to L.I.F.E. Fit, is my inspiration. This book is not only dedicated to you but is thanks to you.

I am so lucky and humbled to have so many people to thank. I owe thanks and gratitude to my friends and family whose patience, endless enthusiasm and encouragement for my work has been unfaltering in the creation of my L.I.F.E. Fit programme, the growth of my business We Fit Together and the writing of L.I.F.E. Fit - The Process. Your support is both inspiring and empowering.

My life, love and eternal appreciation is dedicated to my Husband, Dean who has unknowingly completed me and has provided me with a life that I cherish. Without Dean's belief in me, my work would not have been possible and my L.I.F.E. Fit programme and subsequently this book, would still just be dominating room in my head and not in the hands and minds of Mums, which is where it should be. Thank you, Dean for giving me the opportunity to bring my work to life. Thank you for giving me a security that allows me to breath, to feel happy, safe and loving life. For everything that you do and for everything that you are, thank you.

To my Son Sean, who from the moment you were placed in my arms, has given me a strength to rise tall above all fears and a love that has no boundaries. It is true what they say, "a mother holds her child's hand for a short while and their hearts forever" Whatever we do for our children, I don't think they truly realise what they do for us or the impact they have on our lives. Thank you for being you Sean, keep doing what you are doing.

To my step-sons, Jesse and Kalan, who have taught me that maternal love and the want to protect are not emotions borne from biology alone. Thank you both for accepting me into your lives.

To my grandparents, thank you for everything!

"Your life is what you make it, make your life worthwhile. Be happy"
Jean Tunbridge (my Nan)

CONTENTS

EXERCISES EXPLAINED

1

L.I.F.E. FIT – THE PROCESS

how can it help

I am Jessica Revell, I am a fitness and weight loss coach training my clients to lose weight, drop body fat and tone up, using my L.I.F.E. Fit programme to create beautifully lean, feminine bodies. I created my L.I.F.E. Fit programme as it became more and more apparent that we mums need more than just an exercise routine and meal plan to help us overcome the differing emotions we seem to bounce between. These emotions often get in the way and hamper any success of a body transformation, but seem to come hand in hand with being a mum and there is no getting around them.

There are many weight loss plans and programmes available, all of them providing you with an exercise schedule and meal plan to follow and these are great, if you haven't got children to consider as well as yourself. As weight loss programmes are so often designed for one person to follow exclusively, it is an almost impossible task to implement and to fully benefit from in the long term when you are trying to incorporate them into an already packed day. L.I.F.E. Fit - The Process is a series of simple principles within my L.I.F.E. Fit programme, meaning that with this book, I can now bring the many benefits of my L.I.F.E. Fit Programme to Mums and their families everywhere.

As mums, we often want to lose the baby weight, to tone up for the next family holiday, or to lose the weight accumulated over the years of family dinners and children's birthday parties. We all want to get a flat stomach and look sculpted in our bikinis. But as mums, our health and fitness needs are actually more complex than they were before our children came along. We have more to consider than just ourselves and deeper emotions to deal with now; whether you are a mum with young children and have found yourself at home for the first time rather than in the office with your work friends, and you are struggling to maintain your own identity, or whether you are the mum with older children and you are trying to get through the hot flushes and hormonal changes and you need to keep control of your body, there are now many more aspects to consider when talking about losing weight, getting fit and being healthy.

Whilst thinking about how we can regain a toned, feminine body, we are at the same time worrying about how we can make sure our children grow up healthy, both physically and emotionally. As well as thinking about what we should and shouldn't be eating and what exercises we should be doing to stay fit, as mums we are also concerned about making sure our children are eating enough of what they need. We have the worry of making sure our children are as active as they should be. We worry about our children's emotions and whether they know they have a friend in us as well as being 'just their mum'. We worry about our children developing a negative body image and at the same time as trying to keep control of our own weight, we must ensure that our efforts do not impose a negative attitude towards food in our children. As mums, we experience these emotions on top of our concerns about our weight, our dress size and body shape. So how do we, as mums, successfully follow a programme that will give us weight loss results, tone our bodies and increase our health whilst simultaneously providing a healthy upbringing for our children leading to positive attitudes towards food and exercise as they grow older?

Being a mum doesn't mean you need to stop being you. There is a way to stay in control of your life and be in control of your body, to be fit and healthy and at the same time be confident about your children's physical and emotional wellbeing. It is just a case of following a little Process.... The Process!

My L.I.F.E. Fit programme has transformed the mind-set and bodies of mums up and down the country, bringing health and fitness into the homes of mums with new babies, with toddlers, with young children and with teenagers. As well as losing weight and toning their bodies, each person who followed The Process improved their bodies, their fitness, their health and most importantly of all, introduced a healthy lifestyle throughout their home. A lifestyle that would go on to improve the lives of their children, who are now growing up in an environment where health and fitness is a way of life; a normal routine that they are simply growing up with. Healthy, nutritious food is something that is enjoyed by the whole family together and where exercise is a fun family activity.

What has driven you to read this book? What is it that you are looking to improve? Maybe you want to improve your health, maybe you want to increase your fitness, to lose weight, to tone up, to build muscle definition? Let's start this book as we mean to go on and keep it honest. We all know you can pick up any home fitness DVD and choose from an abundance of new and improved diet and clean eating books, using them to start a new routine that will help you on your way to any of the above. And many of them I am sure will work for a lot of Mums, giving some results... initially at least. Unfortunately, most home fitness programmes available are aimed at one individual to follow and do not take family life into account, giving meal ideas for one person and recipes that adults may like but that most children will generally turn their nose up at. This ultimately leads to you following the programme for a while, cooking the healthy meals on the meal plan for yourself and then having to cook separate meals for everyone else in the family. So, the question here is, if the meals you are feeding your children are healthy meals.... Why are you not able to eat them too? And if your children's' meals are not healthy enough for you to eat, why are your children being given them to eat? So, as a Mum who wants to lose weight and drop dress sizes and who has children to consider in everything she does, what should a weight loss programme for mums really deliver?

- to get back control of our lives and to regain our identity
- to lose unwanted body fat and maintain the weight loss for the long term
- to feel in control of our bodies
- to feel in control of our children's health and emotional wellbeing
- to know that we are bringing our children up in a healthy environment.
- to generally feel good about ourselves!

By following L.I.F.E. Fit - The Process, you can achieve all of this and your own body transformation is simply a natural side effect.

So here you are, running your home with your children in tow; can you remember the time when you had a name other than 'mum'? A time when nipping out of the house to go to the gym or for a run or to simply take a walk was no more complicated than throwing your trainers on? Now, even if your children are at school, you must squeeze these times into a schedule of meal planning, homework, washing, cleaning, school runs, shopping, tantrums, the list goes on. For those of you who have gone back to work after having your children, well that's just another something to deal with, something else eating into your limited time.

Don't get me wrong, being a mum is a privileged position and brings with it many rewards but all privileged positions do come with their drawbacks. In this case, how much of yourself have you lost as you spend your days running around looking after everyone else? How much time have you spent on *you* as you decide each day what to cook your family for dinner, or when the weekly shop should get done? Or whether enough shirts have been ironed for the week...? Do you remember pre-children when you had the time and opportunity to dress up every day; to make an effort with your hair and make-up and you could walk around feeling good about yourself? This opportunity doesn't happen so much when your daily routine barely allows time for a coffee stop; your polished pre-children look has been taken over by scrunched-back hair, jeans and pumps. You dash around on the school runs and in between tidy the house, wash the clothes, put baby down for a nap, do the grocery shopping, take the children to the park and soft play centres, become taxi driver, plan, prepare and cook breakfast, lunch and dinner, and for a lot of you squeeze in a job too. How much of your time is spent on *you*? How much of your time, running around doing all your tasks, is actually spent as real one-on-one time with your children where they have your undivided attention, just you and them? It is all too easy to follow a routine day after day and before you know it, your babies grow into toddlers, your toddlers turn into children, your children stop relying on you as much as they become more independent and your teenagers are like passing ships in the night. You have been so busy being 'mum' you didn't have time to stop and take it all in, to enjoy it. Your children grow up fast and you are often too busy to really see it happening. While all of this is going on, you have been so busy being thrown from one day to the next you didn't notice your own clothes getting tighter and any new clothes that you buy getting bigger. You have been so busy being 'mum' you forgot about *you*, and without even knowing when, you have realised that you aren't confident in your own body any more. Your self-esteem has dropped and you have lost a part of your own identity. The irony of this is, the very routine that put you in this position is the same routine that now leaves you too tired to do anything about it. More to the point, maybe you tried to do something about it, choosing a programme designed to help individuals rather than parents and as a result found it too difficult to implement with any success and gave up, believing that you can't do anything about it.

My mission is to help mums realise just how easy it can be to take back control of their lives, to re-establish who they are over and above being 'mum' and to get their body back into a shape that gives them the confidence and self-esteem that often diminishes with each dirty nappy, sleepless night, terrible twos tantrum and teenagers' meltdown.

Over and above this, it is my mission to help mums realise that health and fitness does not have to be a solo activity and certainly shouldn't isolate you from everyone else in your family, especially at meal times. On the contrary, L.I.F.E. Fit - The Process will show you that food and exercise are actually fantastic interests to share with your children and that your children will love sharing with you. Most importantly of all, L.I.F.E. Fit - The Process will show you that your weight loss journey is not something that you need to stress or obsess over. L.I.F.E. Fit - The Process will show you how to approach your weight loss and healthy lifestyle without turning your life upside down. You will never need to concern yourself with another trendy FAD diet again! This book will concentrate on you as the mum, but it will soon become apparent how following The Process will bring health and fitness into your home while you lose weight, tone up and get fit... surely that is a winning combination!

Being a mum myself, I am very much aware that our daily routines are for the benefit of our children, for the house, for the family and there is no 5.30pm finish. Being a mum is more than a full-time job! A mum generally puts everyone and everything before herself and our daily task list is endless. So, when then, is a mum supposed to prioritise her needs? Where is the time to even think about weight loss and exercise plans, nutritious meals and family together times? I created The Process specifically for the mum:

- who wants to do something for herself, but not at the expense of time with her children
- who wants to take control back of her life
- who wants her body back and wants to look toned and feminine but who does not want to spend hours a day exercising or have a restricted, complicated diet to follow
- Who wants to follow a realistic programme that takes into account the health and wellbeing of everyone in the family home
- Who wants a programme that understands the demands of being a Mum and works to enhance family life rather than add extra pressure to it

My L.I.F.E Fit programme has been created to help mums achieve all of this and more. L.I.F.E. Fit - The Process will create a healthy routine that will spread throughout the house, benefiting the children as well as the parents. It will introduce nutrition and exercise into your house, creating a healthy lifestyle for you and your family whilst making way for new bonding times between you and your children. The principles within this book will ultimately create a state of physical health and emotional well-being that will benefit every child and adult within the home.

Using a strong unity between food, eating patterns and exercise, L.I.F.E. Fit - The Process has proven time and time again to create happy, healthy and fit households up and down the country. By following the L.I.F.E. Fit principles your household can also experience the powerful family health and fitness benefits. You will burn body fat and achieve your weight loss goals as you sculpt a toned, feminine body, while your children will benefit from your new healthy lifestyle as you all create realistic family routines.

2

INTRODUCTION

what is L.I.F.E. Fit - The Process

EVERYBODY has the power to change. Whether you recognise this in yourself or not, no matter who you are, no matter what you do, if you want it you can make it.

If you are holding this book and flicking through its pages it is because you are looking for answers; you know you want to change your body, you know you want to start a healthier way of life with good food and exercise. You know you want your children to benefit from a healthy lifestyle. Maybe you recognise that you have lost a little of your own identity, lost a little control over your own life, and you want to re-establish who you are since having children. You know you want all of this and you want to know how you can achieve it. Maybe you are wondering if any of this really is possible.

The majority of my clients started with a desire to transform their bodies, to lose weight, to tone up and to get fit. As well as wanting to look good, this desire to start a new weight loss programme is often the first step most mums take in re-establishing themselves and to regain control. So, the big question is, can a mum who rushes around with no time to spare really undertake a programme that will be successful in creating a body transformation?

The answer is simple…. YES! And what's more, it doesn't take hours in the gym. It doesn't mean having nothing but cabbage or juice forever and it doesn't mean finding a babysitter or nursery every time you exercise. This book will not lead you to follow some new fad diet. It will not list some long, overcomplicated and highly restricted food plan and it will not ask you to exercise for hours every day. On the contrary, The Process will see you following healthy eating and exercise habits that will not only benefit you, but which your children will grow to see as normal, daily activities too. We teach our children by example, and thus the habits and routines they witness as they grow up will hopefully be the same habits and routines they themselves will go on to follow in adulthood, and will naturally include in their daily lives. It is the start of a new, healthy life cycle.

As you follow L.I.F.E. Fit - The Process it will teach you how your body needs to be fed and moved. The principles within this book will get your body burning excess body fat and will transform your body to be tight, lean and toned. L.I.F.E. Fit - The Process will start your body burning fat so effectively you will be amazed by the changes you see. What's more, by following L.I.F.E. Fit's principles you will learn that your exercise time can be at any time during the day and done anywhere. Your children can get involved, be your coach or simply watch; either way, you will be introducing fun activities and challenges into your home that your children will want to be a part of, and therefore they too will be benefiting. Over and above this, without any effort, you will be creating quality, uninterrupted time with your children, regardless of whether they are toddlers, young children or teenagers and as your children get older, they in turn will naturally want to involve you in their sporting and fitness activities as much as they were involved in yours.

By continuing to read this book you will be taken through each surprisingly simple stage, leading you to a complete body transformation and a whole new healthy lifestyle for you and your family.

Now, the fundamentals of L.I.F.E. Fit - The Process will focus on you as the Mum. It will concentrate on your own weight loss and the principles you need to follow to get your own body burning fat and dropping dress sizes. Follow these principles and everything else will fall into place. So, for the remainder of this book, let's talk about you and concentrate on putting you back in control.

As a mum, you will look at your new baby, your young children and your fast-growing teenagers with so much love and pride. You worry constantly about their health, about whether you are giving them the right foods, about making sure they are active enough. Well, everything has a starting point and to ensure your children have a healthy life and grow up living an active and healthy lifestyle, guess what…. You are that starting point. You can preach to your children until you are blue in the face about what they should be eating and how they should be outside instead of indoors on their smartphone or tablet but the truth is, children will only learn from example. By that I mean, until they see you, their mum setting examples as a normal daily routine, no amount of preaching will have an impact on them. So, it is time to do something for yourself and learn the principles of L.I.F.E. Fit - The Process.

If you can have pride in yourself and feel good about how you look, imagine how other people will see you. Imagine how your children will see you. Imagine how good you will feel about yourself knowing your children are proud of how you look. Imagine how good you will feel to be the mum who looks fantastic and confident and more than anything else, in control. So, if I said to you, your whole family can enjoy being healthy together but we need to concentrate on transforming your body and making you confident in yourself.... Would you be interested?

I am a mum who through self-experience, test groups and client success stories can honestly say to you, follow L.I.F.E. Fit - The Process and like me and all my clients, you WILL lose body fat, you WILL tone up and you WILL feel and look amazing ... oh and your whole family will be healthy as a result...!

Just imagine having enough energy to enjoy your family. To have a body that you feel good in. Imagine opening your wardrobe every morning and being able to ask yourself "what do I WANT to wear today?" rather than "what CAN I wear today?"

You will not need to dedicate yourself to hours of exercise to make this work and L.I.F.E. Fit – The Process does not say 'never eat' to any foods. It allows for real life and makes that a real healthier life. It gives you control back and it delivers real results.

I know it is everyone's dream to have that 'perfect' body and just because we are now mums, does not mean we lose that desire to have a good body. Whatever your idea of 'perfect' is and wherever you are starting this journey from, whatever your current weight, size or age please remember one thing... don't wait to reach your weight loss goals before you acknowledge your beauty. Enjoy your weight loss journey and believe that you are already beautiful! It is as important for your children to see you happy in yourself as it is for your own wellbeing to feel happy in yourself. I know we all dream of having a shapely toned body with a lifted pert butt, flat stomach and lean legs and for some, this body type may have come easy in your pre-children years and you are now on quest to get yourself back to where you were. Or maybe you have never felt good in your body. Maybe you have never had the confidence to wear a bikini, choosing instead to hit the beach covering up in a swimsuit or even avoiding the beach all together. This was how I used to be. I would be the one sitting on the beach on holiday in 32 degrees' heat in a swimsuit and sarong, covering as much of my body up as possible. I would watch the other women on the beach in their bikinis, looking as if they didn't have a care in the world and wishing I could look like that. I would dread the summer months knowing that I would feel uncomfortable and very self-conscious in the long clothes that I used to hide my body in. Can you relate to that? Have you ever walked along your local high street in the summer feeling like the only person who doesn't look sexy? Seeing all the other women in their shorts and strappy tops and wishing you could wear the same? You can.... you absolutely can, mums are sexy too! By following L.I.F.E. Fit - The Process you really can be healthy, strong, fit and sexy. You can wear your summer clothes and you can feel confident on the beach. You can do this and still be able to eat real food. You don't need to eat separately from your children, or cook yourself different meals from everyone else in the house. No matter what size you are now, or how much you weigh, if you are willing to follow the principles within this book entirely, you will lose body fat and drop dress sizes and you will soon be choosing to wear your favourite summer clothes and be confident in them. Honestly, I have seen the results for myself and time and time again on my clients.

So, imagine now looking and feeling tight, toned and graceful in your movements. Imagine having energy levels that keep you going all day without having the tiredness in the afternoon. Imagine having a body that feels lean and defined and looks as good you feel.

- The Process is the start of your journey where this is all possible without making food your enemy.
- The Process is your beginning to a way of life where food is not a struggle and where physical fitness is a natural occurrence and not a laughable dream or dread.
- The Process is a way of life where your clothes slip on and feel comfortable whatever you choose to wear

This really is achievable. I am a Mum and had the same struggles and it worked for me and over years of research and testing it has worked for my clients with one, two, three and even four children who each followed my L.I.F.E. Fit programme and achieved the results that they each desired. The baby pouch flattened, the bloated stomach gone, the legs toned and the butt lifted and tightened. It really is possible! And what's more, this was all achieved by never entering a gym or learning how to cook complicated recipes with unpronounceable ingredients. I promise you, no matter what made you pick this book up, no matter what your current weight is or what your current size is, whatever your personal story is, as long as you follow the L.I.F.E. Fit principles completely and consistently, it will work for you. All you have to do is trust The Process!

We all have our own personal story leading us to look for weight loss answers. We can all sit down and trace back to establish at what point our lives became so hectic we lost control of any manageable routine. Are you the mum with three beautiful children and a stomach you hide every day? Are you the mum who goes to the gym every day and puts everything you have into a group class, but with no noticeable results to speak of? Are you the mum that works all day and runs around after your children all night?

Over the years working with my clients I have heard many varying personal stories. Everyone has their own personal account of how they got to where they are now. How the weight increased and the dress sizes followed. However, when it comes to losing weight there is one common theme that many mums share: not enough time; not enough time to cook fresh foods. Not enough time to exercise. Not enough time to eat properly. I understand that. Time is short anyway but as soon as you add children to the equation time really is not on our side. What I found even more shocking and in so many cases, actually upsetting was to hear the stories of how so many of my clients attempted so many shocking methods to lose their weight; the liquid diets that leaves you feeling so hungry you end up eating more than you used to at the beginning and as a result feel even worse about yourself than you did at the start. The mums that are so desperate to look amazing and to be the 'yummy mummy' they see in the celebrity magazines that they starve themselves, leaving their meals in replacement for water, coffee or tea, all in a scary attempt to be tiny. The mental self-abuse we women torment ourselves with just because we simply want to look good and like what we see in the mirror is unbelievable but all too common. The saddest part of these weight loss attempts is not only the damage they cause to your own body and mental well-being but the message these diet cycles have on our children. What lessons are we teaching them by following these ridiculous yo-yo dieting routines? How can we expect our children to grow up to have a healthy relationship with food and a confident body image if all they have seen while growing up are the diet battles they saw you experience throughout their childhood? It is important to remember that the actions you are seen to take and the habits you are seen to follow are the actions and the habits that your children, no matter how young or old, will grow up to follow themselves. Following dangerous 'diet' rules is just as bad for your body, health and fitness as is eating too much and more often than not is the very thing that will lead you to eat too much. If you want your children to grow up with healthy habits, they must see you following healthy habits. It is as damaging for your children to witness parents overeating the wrong foods and living a sedentary lifestyle as it is seeing their parents over-exercising and obsessing about losing more weight. Both ends of the scale can cause damaging, long lasting effects on our children's own body image and own battles with food later in their own adult life.

L.I.F.E. Fit - The Process is not about restricting your food to impossibly low levels, nor is it about cooking long, complicated recipes or exercising for hours each day and it is certainly not about some 'quick fix' dangerous weight loss method. L.I.F.E. Fit - The Process is about balance, it is about creating healthy lifestyles that are realistic and achievable for families to maintain. The principles of L.I.F.E. Fit are surprisingly simple but remarkably powerful!

I created my L.I.F.E. Fit programme for many accumulating reasons. Initially because I have been through the torment of hating my body. I have felt the desperation of wanting to make the change in my body but not knowing where to turn or what to do to make that change. I was constantly baffled by the overwhelming choice of home DVD programmes to follow and still remained confused about what I should be doing with food. I then recognised the same battles in other women and knew it was time for something better. Something that actually got results and something that is accessible to everyone, achievable by everyone, and more importantly, something that works in real family life. I created my L.I.F.E. Fit programme because I recognised that as a mum, anything I did now would be what my children would in turn grow to do themselves, and that the lifestyle I led had to be the lifestyle I wanted for my children. The examples I set in my home now are what would influence my children's future, and that is what drove me forward. L.I.F.E. Fit - The Process not only delivers body changing results for you as a mum, but puts you in control of your own state of mind and your children's physical and mental well-being. So now is the time to ask yourself:

- Do you want to change your body?
- Do you want to be fit and toned?
- Do you want to be full of energy?
- Do you want more self-confidence?
- Do you want to reinvent the way your body looks and moves?
- Do you want your children to grow up healthy and fit?

The solution is simple. Continue reading this book. Follow its principles and trust The Process!

3

JESSICA'S STORY

why I created L.I.F.E. Fit

I know what it is like to feel uncomfortable in your own body. I know how it feels to look in the mirror and hate your own reflection. I know what it feels like to feel absolute desperation to want to feel smaller and tighter but have no idea how to achieve it. I know how it feels to follow a diet plan and still not see the weight coming off permanently. From an early age, I knew that I needed to exercise more and eat better but never really knew how to exercise or what to eat and more to the point *when* to eat.

I had an increasing desperation to lose weight and to be smaller, and a growing frustration with the lack of definite answers or any form of real direction from the fitness world. There were thousands of different exercise programmes and different 'diets' to follow (and I have tried them all) but nothing that really worked. Once I found an exercise programme to work with I still had to find a diet to match. There was nothing out there that really told me how to exercise effectively and how to eat in conjunction with those exercises. Consequently, I would follow an exercise programme for a while and restrict my food levels to a point where I had no energy and a raging hunger. Ultimately and unavoidably, this would lead to the same result; no energy to exercise and a hunger that led me to eating even more, and so I would be left unmotivated and disillusioned, believing that it was my body type that stopped me from losing weight. I doubted myself, believing that nothing I tried would work, and I would sink further into self-doubt, desperation and frustration.

My weight and how to lose it became a daily battle. I would ask myself, why am I not losing weight? What do I have to do to lose fat? Why are these exercises not working for me? Why is this diet not making me smaller? I developed a real resentment of food, fearful of everything I ate. At that time, I did not recognise the real connection between exercising and eating. There was nothing that explained how to exercise for long term results and nothing that explained *how* to eat. There was nothing available that explained to me what the body needed to function properly other than the usual 'eat your five a day' advice, which to be honest didn't really provide the information I needed. There was nothing to tell me how to feed the body to make it work to its full ability and how it needed to be moved to sculpt the body effectively. More to the point, there was nothing available that explained how to do all of these in tandem to get my body working to its full capacity. Not having these answers, and knowing that, once obtained, they would give me the golden solution for weight loss and body transformation, was the catalyst in my journey. The realisation that this is what I needed to know to achieve my weight loss is what threw me into a new desperation; a desperation to *learn*.

I needed to know everything about the workings of our bodies. What fuelled it and how. How the muscles were developed and how they needed to be moved. I finally realised that it was not my fault that I had failed every diet I'd tried but that the direction and information simply wasn't there for me, for anyone really in the general public!

This was the start of my journey. If I could feed my body in the way it is intended to be fed and move my body in a way that sculpted the muscles and burned fat at the same time, then surely, I would be able to transform my body in a way that I had only dreamed of before. If I could do this, then surely everyone could, regardless of body type. It was purely a case of establishing what our bodies needed in order to function. I was so excited that these answers could actually be the key to successful weight loss and body transformations. Now I knew what information I needed, I could start to find out what I really needed to be doing.

Now, to fully appreciate what drove me to this point and what motivated me throughout the following years of research and testing to develop my L.I.F.E Fit programme, you need to understand me and to know my story.

I spent my early years in Leigh on Sea in Essex, where I had a very happy childhood, enjoying my Primary School years immensely. I was the youngest of three children (at the time) with an older brother and an older sister (I now have a younger brother too). My Nan and Granddad lived close by and we would have our Friday night dinner there; fish fingers, chips and beans followed by sweets or chocolate. The last weekend of the month was our sleepover nights at Nan and Granddads.

My Nan was a typical Nan. She always made sure her grandchildren were well fed and watered. I can't remember Nan saying 'No' to too many requests; "Nan can I have an ice cream please? Nan, can I have some penny sweets please? Nan, can I have a glass of coke please?" you get the idea. The food was plentiful. On Sunday mornings, we would get up to a full English breakfast or 3 slices of thick white toast with butter and jam or a large bowl of cereals with full fat milk. This was the breakfast Nan gave us before the whole family would go to a restaurant for a three course Sunday lunch. This was my Nan and Granddad's treat to the family, every last Sunday of the month.

At home, we had a larder full of sweets. Not just any old sweets but large trade size containers of sweets that my Granddad would buy from the cash and carry. I would get home from school grab a selection of sweets for me and my friends and go out to play. The summer months were the best; my friends and I playing out on the street (it was the eighties when it was normal for children to play up and down their street with their friends), running in and out of each other's houses, planning what we would do the next day or at the weekend. Tonibell, the ice cream van would come around every night (usually just before dinner, sometimes straight afterwards). My mum would come out and we would get our Oyster or double Ninety-Nine. I loved summer evenings as a child. That was until I started getting bigger and bigger.

Over the passing years, I was getting bigger than any of my friends. As we reached the latter years of primary school my friends were getting more and more into fashion and makeup. I was too, the difference was I couldn't enjoy it. My friends would come around wearing the rah-rah skirt we had all been talking about at school and the little off the shoulder tops we saw our favourite pop idols wearing and I would be in my baggy t-shirt and oversized culottes. I couldn't wear anything else without feeling uncomfortable. I grew more and more self-conscious and more and more uncomfortable. I couldn't understand why out of all my friends, I was the one who was fat. My parents would always try to control my eating but as a child, I didn't understand the connection between food and body fat. My friends never judged me but I did. I hated how I felt. I was so ashamed of how I looked.

New Years' Eve was always a big family party for us. My grandparents, aunties, uncles and cousins would all come around and we would get dressed up ready for the party in the evening. My sister would always look amazing in her pipeline trousers and silk shirts and I would be the fat little sister resembling the circus tent in my silk shirt.

The day that will stick in my throat forever; we were at school and the teacher took out the weighing scales, then called everyone in the class up one by one to the front of the classroom and weighed us. I felt sick to the core. When it was my turn I walked to the front of the room. My head was down but I felt like everyone was staring at me. I didn't show it but I felt like crying, I felt like running as far away from the room as possible but I didn't. I stood on the scales and held my breath for what must have been seconds but felt like an eternity. The result of this exercise, other than making me feel like the biggest freak in Essex, was my Mum making an appointment for me to visit a dietician. Over the following months, I followed the dietician's plan (or rather my Mum and Nan followed the plan, giving me the foods I was allowed to eat) and the weight did fall off. I was free again to look like the pretty little girl my parents always told me I was. I remember wearing a little short sleeved pink dress with a skirt to my knees and I felt like all my friends; I felt normal.

However, it became very apparent that I certainly did not have the genetic make-up that permitted easy weight control. The following years saw my weight fluctuate dramatically and my high school years was a constant battle with my weight; spending half my time feeling larger than everyone else and wishing I could control my body size.

When I was 13 I moved to Yorkshire with my Mum. My parents had long separated by this point and several chapters of our lives had passed; my Granddad had passed away leaving a huge hole in our lives and my Mum had enrolled in Huddersfield University. We moved to Hyde Park in Leeds and my Nan soon followed. My sister went to Warwick University and my brother joined the army. I started a new school and made new friends. I was many miles away from my Essex home and anything of any familiarity but my battle with my own body continued; I tried not eating, surely if I wasn't eating I couldn't put weight on...right? Wrong, I would get so hungry it wasn't long before I was eating so much of whatever I could get my hands on quickest. So, to prevent the hunger I would live on food replacement pills, sitting in the school canteen swallowing appetite suppressants while my friends tucked into their school lunches. Surely that had to work, right? Wrong again. I was at a loss. I did not know what to do. I could lose weight and keep it off for a while then it would creep back on again and I couldn't track why. And so this is how my teenage years went on. Sometimes I would feel good about myself but in large, I was overweight and bigger than I wanted to be.

I discovered dance in high school. Other than ballet and tap dance in primary school, this was the first time I really felt my body move in a way that made me feel the closest to elegant as I ever had before. I could lose myself in the music and I felt light on my feet. Dance became my release over the years and was my introduction to exercise and body movement. As long as the music was playing I could move my body. I went on to use music to dance to, to run to, to exercise to and as I discovered all the different things I could do with my body, I went on to lift weights too. I had never felt as good about myself as I did at this point. I was finally at ease with how I looked most of the time. I say most of the time because I still had to work so hard to maintain my new size. I had to be so careful with food and if I so much as looked at a chip my hips would increase in size. Obviously not literally but the point is that is how I felt. So, was I really free? Not really. Yes, I was smaller but I was still having daily battles with food in order to maintain my smaller frame. I was exercising for over an hour in the morning and running 5 miles an evening and still felt that I should be doing more.

By now I was in my twenties and my life had seen many transitions. By this time, I was living and working in Harrogate, North Yorkshire. I had what I believed to be an amazing job, working with incredible people. I had continued my routine of going to the gym every morning before work and either running, Yoga, playing badminton or swimming every evening after work. I enjoyed my exercise routine but still had to be so careful with my food and yes, my body was certainly smaller and more toned than I had been in my earlier years but I still wanted to see a more drastic result for the work I was putting in.

This all came to a sudden stop however when a silly accident resulted in me breaking my neck. When squatting with 60KG across my neck I lost my footing, falling flat on my bum with the 60kg bar landing across my neck, breaking the C1 and C2 vertebrae. I could have had an operation to try to fix the damage but I was told that the operation carried a 70% chance of paraplegia as they would have had to have operated dangerously close to my spinal cord. The following months were spent in bed with a heavy dose of pain management through 12 hourly doses of morphine. The pain lessened over time and 6 months later another scan showed that the vertebra had repaired itself in a way that would still allow an almost full range of neck movement and that the mucoprotein gel that had previously wrapped itself around my spinal cord, trapping many nerves to the upper left-hand side of my body had retracted and was no longer a danger. Dancing, running or any high impact

21

motion was certainly out of the question for the foreseeable future but to be honest, at this stage I was grateful to be walking.

My extended time away from work meant I had to leave my job but this enabled me to build my strength up gradually and it wasn't too long before I was lucky enough to start a new job. Life was almost normal again. I was certainly smaller now but this was because I had spent the past six months on morphine and very little food had been eaten. It wasn't a small, fit frame that I had now, it was a weak body but I certainly wasn't in a hurry to start exercising at this point. I think this was the first time that I had stopped obsessing about my body. I spent the next year simply being. Obviously, I watched what I ate (carefully) and I walked as often as possible but I didn't enter a gym. I couldn't go running and for some reason I didn't beat myself up over it.

Whether it was a reaction to the accident and recovery time or whether it was because other events in my life were dominating my very being but either way something in me had changed, I had lost a little spark in me. Even a year later I still had no desire to dance, no drive to exercise and although I continued to be conscious about food, as the months passed, I started caring less and less about what I ate.

I loved living and working in the beautiful spa town of Harrogate but this wasn't a happy time in my life. This was a dark chapter and I was (or felt) powerless to change things. All that said though, this was also the time when I was about to embark on the scariest but most exciting and rewarding part of my life so far. I started going to the shops mid-morning driven by a need for biscuits. I would bring back a selection of biscuits for the office and find myself eating most of them. I started to feel a hunger I had never felt before; I didn't fancy a biscuit.... I *needed* a biscuit. Not just one, but one after another after another. All you mum's reading this can surely guess what was happening.... yes, I was pregnant. Can you remember that feeling when you found out you were pregnant? Scared, excited, overwhelmed.

When you found out that you were pregnant, what was your initial thought process? Did your body shape and how it will change occur to you? Did it bother you to think that you will get bigger and that once your new baby was born you will be left with weight to lose? I was concerned by this but to be honest, and contrary to how I had spent my life so far, my body shape and any excess weight were not key factors during my pregnancy. I did join an aqua fit class and I did try to eat healthily most of the time but this was predominantly for the benefit of my baby more than anything else.

I went through my pregnancy with no health problems and at the time was very happy that I did not actually get too big during those months. Yes, obviously I got bigger but I did not really start looking pregnant until halfway through the third trimester. On the 30th October 2004 Sean, my perfect baby boy was born and I got to hold all 5lb 13oz of him. I was immediately besotted with him.

Sean was born at 12.50am and at 5.30pm Sean and I were sent home. I can remember getting ready to leave the hospital and putting on a pair of jeans that were not maternity jeans and feeling very smug with myself. My body had survived a pregnancy without too much damage. I shouldn't have been so smug. It was the following months that would see my baby weight creep on.

I had chosen to breastfeed. As a first- time mum I wanted to try breastfeeding anyway but also, I had been told that the act of breastfeeding promotes your stomach muscles to knit back together. I must admit that this was a factor in my choice.

And so my new baby routine started. This would see me eating…. lots; crisps, chocolates, pasties. I would have breakfast, lunch and dinner and plenty of snacks in between. I felt the weight going back on and it wasn't long before the all too familiar feelings of self-consciousness started kicking in. The weight piled on and the jeans I wore to come home from hospital in no longer fitted. I couldn't even pull them up. My size just increased and although I saw and felt it happening, I couldn't (or didn't) do anything about it. As the first year passed, Sean was growing fast... and so was I. Things were still not working out for me in Yorkshire and with a new-found strength in me since having Sean I moved back to my home town of Southend, where I would start my new life as a single mum.

It felt strange to be back in Essex but events in my life had taken me to rock bottom and coming home to Southend was the start of my long climb back to the top. On top of everything else, my old friend desperation had come back to visit, and all the questions about my weight and how to lose it that I had all those years before had returned. What exercises should I be doing? What should I be eating? How should I be exercising? This time however, perhaps learning from my younger years, I decided not to spend all my time in the gym. Apart from anything else, I had a baby now, I couldn't go to the gym for an hour every morning before going to work and I certainly couldn't go running every evening. I had a baby to look after and a life to rebuild. I didn't want my weight issues to consume my life. I didn't want to fall into the trap of trying every trending fitness routine and fad diet. This time, as well as thinking about me and my own health and weight loss, I had Sean's health to consider. This time I wasn't just an overweight woman. I was an overweight mum and any new routine that I embarked on had to benefit me and my son. The foods that were cooked at home had to be the right foods and be healthy as I was solely responsible for Sean's wellbeing now. I had to ensure that as a growing child, Sean could enjoy daily physical activity as well as making sure I got my daily exercise done. This was all new to me, I had only ever had myself to consider before now and to be honest, being solely responsible for a child's health can be somewhat overwhelming, especially when you have spent your whole life trying to understand your own health needs. As I spent my days between work, soft play centres and toddler groups I was amazed to see that so many other women were fighting the same battles as I was; battles with their own bodies, battles with knowing what to eat and what their children should be eating. This was not a unique problem, it was everywhere. It was not only me who was affected by this constant body battle; every mum I spoke to or overheard had the same body weight anxieties as I did, the same fight to be slim and the same struggles to find the information about real weight loss. Every mum was asking the same questions and shared the same concerns: how can I exercise with baby at home? I'm too tired to exercise; what meals should I be eating; what food should my children be having...? It was then that I realised there must be answers out there, and that I had to find them. I realised that I had to approach my own weight loss differently this time. I realised that for my son to live a healthy life, he had to live in a healthy home, and that could only come about if I made it a healthy home. I couldn't expect my son to grow up with a healthy relationship with food and a good body confidence if he constantly saw me battling with my weight and obsessing about food. I understood now the importance of my role as 'Mum' I knew this time I had to get it right. I had to learn everything about our bodies and what they needed to be fit and healthy. No more cycles of over-eating and starving myself, no more over exercising or silly fad diets or quick fixes. I needed to know what the body needed in terms of food and how the body needed to be moved. I had an example to set and I had to know how to do it properly. So, this time I researched!

I wanted to know everything about the body and what it really needed in terms of food and activity. I wasn't interested in the fad diets that everyone was trying, or the latest celebrity weight loss trend. This time, I wanted the truth, the science. I had to learn about how the body is energised through food and how physical activity uses this energy. I needed to know about the effects of nutrients and how the body reacts differently to different exercises. I found out how different movements affected different muscle groups and how each muscle needed to be moved to sculpt and shape them. I learned how our muscles worked and how they could be changed. It soon became very apparent that there was a lot of information out there about weight lifting and building muscle but this was always shown to be very masculine and intimidating. There was also plenty of cardio workout DVDs and these all looked very feminine and seemed to concentrate more on coordination and choreography than they did on effective cardio work. There was nothing that showed how to best combine the two. Nothing that showed women how to use weights effectively or cardio that was effective in burning fat. It was at this point I started writing my own exercise programmes. I was beginning to understand what I needed to be doing to shape my body how I wanted it. I was beginning to see that any successful weight loss and body transformation had to incorporate body and weight resistance to strengthen and form muscle mass together with effective cardio to burn body fat. I started developing methods that incorporated weights and high intensity interval training simultaneously. I learned how to move to shape the body and sculpt the muscles whilst burning fat at the same time, in one workout. And by combining these strategic moves while the heart rate was up meant only half the time was required to see results. It was a real eye-opener to see how the simplest of moves put into a specific order could make such a difference to how the body reacts and changes.

I used my own body to test and trial, working through each part of the body. The biggest difference for me this time was that I didn't have the luxury of being able to go to the gym whenever I wanted. I had my son at home with me and any exercise routine I started had to be able to fit seamlessly into my already busy day as a mum. To begin with, I would wait for Sean to be in bed or down for his nap before I worked out because that was the advice that was given; to get your workout done while baby is sleeping. As time passed however and Sean's sleeping patterns changed it was harder to train at nap times because we wouldn't always be at home when Sean napped. Sometimes he would fall asleep in the car, or while shopping. So, rather than waiting for Sean to be asleep before I exercised, I simply just got on with it while Sean was up and playing. I would train with him in the room and this in itself was a learning curve; Sean would choose to watch me exercise rather than watch TV. He would want to help me by timing me and sometimes, he would join in…. well, it was a young child's version of joining in but the point is, as a young child, he showed an interest in physical activity. Not because I had asked him to or because I had set any particular tasks for him but because he had started to see me exercise every day at home and it became 'normal' to him. He started to see them as play times and we would laugh and have fun while I worked out. My workouts became fun sessions for me and my son. An unexpected lesson in my new training routine was the realisation that as time went on, Sean was demonstrating his own acceptance and acknowledgment that physical exercise was a normal part of daily routine.

My research and trial sessions on the exercises were going well, and I felt that I had finally found the answers to the questions that I had grown up with. However, I knew that this was only one part of a successful weight loss programme. I knew that exercising effectively would only work to a degree, and that eating correctly was pivotal to any success. From personal experience, I knew it was pointless following any exercise routine without eating properly. It was the information I discovered when researching this that opened my eyes to my whole approach to food. What I discovered made so much sense and explained why nothing I had ever done before had worked. I was literally shocked by what I was learning. The research papers that showed overwhelmingly how our bodies needed to be fed to function properly and to burn fat changed my perspective on everything.

At last I could make sense of the body. I could understand why all my previous attempts at weight loss hadn't worked and why it wasn't working for so many other women. It was like a light had been switched on. And you know what?! It was so simple. I started eating as our bodies need us to eat, following a pattern that gives the body everything it needs to do what it needs to do. It wasn't a diet. I didn't go without food and I was eating real food that Sean and I liked. Simple family meals that we could eat together rather than cooking one thing for me and something separate for Sean. I wasn't calorie counting, I wasn't allocating a point system to different foods. I was simply eating how the body needed feeding. Honestly,

I could not believe how effective this was, how much body fat I was losing and at how good I finally felt about myself. At last I finally felt in control. I felt in control of my body, in control of what I was eating. I didn't feel like I would put a stone on simply by eating chips. I felt my body shrinking and tightening. At last food didn't control me.

Now, combining the eating patterns with the exercise routines... I could almost cry for not knowing this all those years ago. I wanted everyone to know how to do what I had just done. I needed to know if this would work for everyone. I put together a test group to include mums with one child, mums with two, three and four children, women who had no children, women who had a young baby and women whose youngest child was now a teenager. I included all age groups and all fitness levels. We measured, we weighed, we exercised using my moves and routines and I explained the principles of my eating method, asking the women to follow a specific eating pattern. The results were unquestionable. The weight fell off, the muscles were defined, long and lean and the energy levels were increased. Everyone who followed my L.I.F.E. Fit programme entirely, achieved real body changing results. After all my years of fighting against my own body at last I had figured it out. All along it simply boiled down to a simple process.... The Process.

Now blissfully happy and still living in Southend, married to my wonderful husband Dean, who has unknowingly completed me and brought a happiness to my life that I had only previously dreamed about, and with Sean now 12 years old and every bit his mother's pride I am also lucky enough to have two new additions to my life in the shape of two amazing step sons, Jesse and Kalan. My L.I.F.E. Fit programme is a simple process and now that my life is very much fulfilled and not having any more personal battles to conquer means I can now bring L.I.F.E. Fit- The Process to you.

Everyone can follow the principles of L.I.F.E. Fit - The Process. It has changed the mind-set and the bodies of so many. I will spend the rest of this book explaining how simple the Process is to follow and how amazingly powerful its effects are, and hopefully you will want to read on to find out for yourself. All I can say is please try it. Follow the Principles within this book and see the results for yourself.

4

WHY IT WORKS

the science bit….I will keep this short

OK, let's talk about exercising. Our bodies are marvellous machines and are designed to move in many ways and directions; not just backwards, forwards, up and down and in order to shape and sculpt your body, you need to be moving your body in different ways, using various moves to target different body parts, sometimes with weights, sometimes without weights. My L.I.F.E. Fit programme uses weights to build muscle mass and high intensity interval training cardio to burn body fat. I know a lot of women are concerned about using weights, believing that they will get big and bulky. The truth is as women, we too need to lift weights to shape our body. This does not mean we are going to build a masculine, bulky body. It is actually very difficult for a woman to build a 'body builders' body. She would need to include a good quality 'gains' protein into her diet and follow a very strict diet together with a specific and relentless exercise programme to achieve her results. You see, as women we don't produce enough testosterone or other hormones to develop big muscles. For the rest of us, the weights will simply improve muscle mass and shape your body. So, yes, the exercises that you will be asked to do when following L.I.F.E. Fit - The Process will include weights. These weights will be light enough for you to use in good form (meaning you will be able to lift them correctly without risking injury) but heavy enough to challenge you. By lifting these weights, you will be creating stronger muscles that will not only shape your body but will actually increase your metabolism. You see, the more muscle mass you have, the higher your resting metabolism will be. The higher your resting metabolism is, the more calories you will burn throughout the day, even when you are not exercising. Weights are our friends and you will learn to love them, honestly.

Now, let's talk cardio. There is no getting around it, we do need to incorporate cardiovascular fitness into any fitness programme. Why? Because we will not improve without it; in order to lose fat, we need to burn fat. Now when we say 'burn fat' the body is not literally burning the fat cells. Instead, it is changing them back to energy and this energy is what is being used to get the body through the cardio work. Therefore, the fat cells are being used instead of being stored. Now, it is important to remember that a calorie is simply a measurement of energy. This means the more calories you eat the more energy you are giving your body. If you do not use that energy, it will be kept by the body and stored as fat cells. So, what we are actually doing during cardio work is turning those fat cells back into energy and using them, hence the saying 'burning fat'. The more effective the cardio work is, the more calories will be burned. Cardio work will also improve the health of your heart and the healthier your heart is, the more effective you can perform your cardio. The cardio work you will be asked to do will be done in an anaerobic state. Anaerobic is different from aerobic; aerobic exercise, which I am sure you are all familiar with, such as running, cycling, swimming and such like needs oxygen to be performed, whereas anaerobic exercise, such as body weight resistance or strength training, creates a need for energy that cannot be supplied through oxygen. Instead your body will draw the required energy from stored fat cells and transfer these back to energy to get you through the work. Aerobic exercise can be sustained for longer periods of time, whereas anaerobic exercise cannot be sustained easily. Aerobic exercise helps to keep the heart healthy and anaerobic exercise burns body fat and builds lean muscle. The body must work through the aerobic state to reach its anaerobic state. My workout sessions will have you working through the aerobic state and into intervals in an anaerobic state, before allowing a brief rest before starting the cycle again. This is the most efficient and effective method for burning fat, building lean muscle and creating a tight, toned body, without the need to exercise for hours each day.

To lose weight you need to be burning more calories than you are eating, fact. There is no getting away from that. So, the stronger your cardiovascular fitness is, the more effective your cardio exercise becomes and ultimately you burn more calories. By incorporating my workout sessions into your routine, the calories are not just being burned while you are working out but will continue to burn long after your exercising has finished. This is called the 'after burn' effect. This is known in the fitness industry as excess post-exercise oxygen consumption or EPOC. Many research papers now show that the high intensity interval training that my programmes incorporate, sparks a high 'after burn effect' and resistance training also sparks a great 'after burn effect' Now, bear in mind my programme combines both, in one session. Just imagine the calories that you will be burning during each workout

AND ongoing throughout the day, long after you have finished exercising. Can you now imagine the sort of results that you really can achieve by following L.I.F.E. Fit - The Process?! By combining the cardiovascular work with the muscle resistance work means you are literally burning the fat away from your body to reveal the newly sculpted muscles that are being formed underneath. The result is a strong, feminine body with long, lean and toned muscles.

I have created a series of exercise sessions for this book, for you to follow. Each session will incorporate High Intensity Interval Training, body resistance and weight resistance. There will always be a modified move to follow for those of you just starting out, together with what can be done as you get stronger to increase the intensity.

Each of the sessions lasts for a total of just 20 minutes and will never include weekends. There has always been a myth that to get results you must train for hours every day. Firstly, who has time for that? Secondly, too much exercise actually prevents results. Training too hard really does drain not only your body but your mind as well, and trust me, when you are training it is your mind that plays the pivotal role in your success. Unless you are an athlete and training for a sporting or fitness event, you really don't need to put your body through hours of exercise each day. If you are hauling yourself through gruelling training sessions for an hour plus every day, not only will you be putting your body through unnecessary stress, it won't be long before you become mentally drained and start talking yourself out of training. Training should not dominate your day, it should slot in easily and benefit your day. My exercise routines are designed to give you brief but intense periods of exercise. Exactly the right amount to challenge and change your body. 20 minutes each weekday and you're done. It is intelligent training and it gets results. Weekends are used for your recovery period, which is just as important as your training sessions. The recovery period is when your muscles respond to the challenges you have given them. Without boring you with anatomy, I will explain briefly that to reshape and tone our muscles we must slightly damage the muscle fibres by overloading them and this is what we are doing during training. Your body then has to repair and rebuild these damaged fibres and it only does this when the body is resting. So, your rest days are actually the days where the changes take place. These rest days are vital and must not be missed. So, when it comes to exercising, more is not best. Intelligent and effective training is the only way and this is how you will be training when following L.I.F.E. Fit - The Process. My training sessions can be followed at any time of the day to suit your daily routine. I know it is often said that to get results you need to train first thing in the morning. Well, in real life, this isn't always possible. If you can't get your training done in the morning, don't, simple as that. The important thing is that you do exercise, be it morning, afternoon or evening.

You don't have to think about what exercise you should be doing or how to do it or in what order. All you need to do is follow the exercises provided and do your best every time. Honestly, it is fun! And no matter how much doubt you have in your mind about your ability to exercise, try it. I won't be asking you to perform some ridiculously choreographed routine. In fact, nothing is choreographed at all. All the moves can be done at your own pace. If you try your best every time, you really will be surprised at what you can do in a short amount of time. You will surprise yourself at how quickly your body responds to the challenges and you will soon feel very proud with yourself at how well you can move your body. Honestly, it won't be too long before the results you see really will be the biggest motivation you need to keep going. Make sure you work up a sweat every time and you will know you are doing it right.

Don't forget, you don't have to wait for your children to be out of the way before you exercise. Let them see you work out, let them join in, let them time you, let them climb on you and have fun with it. I spend my days going from one client to another, all of whom have children at home. The younger children love to scramble under mummy as she holds herself in a plank position. Older children love to stand with me and time the intervals, turning into drill sergeants. Each child gets involved in their own way, even if they are simply sitting on the sofa, initially watching what you are doing; the seeds are being sown. Let your children see you keeping fit, let them see you fitting these workouts into your day, let them see you enjoy your training and let them see you buzzing from it afterwards. Even if they are not interested in doing the same routines you do, they will grow up knowing that physical activity is just a normal daily routine. Remember, my workouts are just 20 minutes. You could run a bath and be done before your bath is ready.

Now, moving on to the eating; you have heard me talking about feeding the body how it needs to be fed, and knowing *how* to eat to get the best from your body. Let me explain what I mean by this; One of the worst pieces of advice I have ever been given, and the same advice that is still given now, is to eat little and often throughout the day, grazing on snacks between breakfast, lunch and dinner. I was always told that it was necessary to eat these snacks between meals to maintain the body's metabolism. Well, at the time, not knowing anything about the body's hormones and how these not only work within the body but actually work to control the body, I followed this advice. I now know that it was this very reason that prevented me from losing weight; I was not allowing time for my body to use the energy provided by the previous meal before I was putting more food (which equals more energy) into my body. The result being, rather than my body being given the chance to use the energy from the first meal before more energy is supplied through the snack, it simply transferred it into fat cells and stored it. So, keeping this as simple as possible, you need to allow the body the sufficient amount of time it needs to deal with the energy provided from each meal. The body has a cycle to follow and requires a set amount of time to do what it needs to do with the energy supply from each meal. It is important for you to understand the importance of this cycle. You need to understand the importance and relevance of these L.I.F.E. Fit principles, because if you don't understand the importance of them, you won't think it matters if you don't follow them. That's the biggest part of L.I.F.E. Fit - The Process…. you must follow it to get the results from it.

Now we all know that we need to eat. Food is an unavoidable necessity for us, which is great for me because, as it turns out, I am a real foodie. The problem is not knowing or understanding how much to eat and when to eat it, and this is the key to successful weight loss. There is a hormone within our body that controls our weight; it dictates when we eat, how much we eat and how much energy our body stores and burns; this is the master hormone, Leptin.

Our bodies are immensely clever, more so than any machine; If food becomes scarce over a period of time, the body's metabolism will slow down in order to prevent too much energy from being used, storing as much energy as it can. With a slower metabolism, the body is now burning the energy at a slower rate in a bid to preserve as much energy as possible for as long as possible. The Leptin hormone signals to your brain, telling it when to preserve the body's energy supply in this way. The only way our bodies can store energy is to transfer it into fat and store it within the body. For women, this storage of body fat is normally around our hips and abdomen. So, by cutting your calorie intake to ridiculously low levels in a bid to lose weight, all you have effectively achieved is a reduced metabolism and an increase in body fat. If, and ultimately when food is then eaten, the reduced metabolism will continue to run slower to preserve the newly provided energy, burning the energy at a slower pace and continuing to store more of the energy as fat. This is the body's primeval survival technique, protecting itself against a further starvation period in case food supply is stopped again. This explains why a diet with a dangerously low calorie intake does not work because ultimately all you are doing is slowing your metabolism down. Then, when the diet itself makes you so hungry you reach out for large amounts of food, your metabolism remains too slow to effectively burn the extra energy that you ultimately go on to give it. The result, your body stores a higher level of fat than it did before you started the diet and you end up bigger than you were at the beginning. This is the classic yo-yo dieting cycle and although most us are aware of this cycle, so many still fall victim to it.

Now I am sure you are all familiar with jumping from diet to diet and the problems we all encounter trying to stick to every one of them; the all too powerful food cravings, the need to snack, especially at night, and the constant fight to stop yourself from reaching for the biscuit tin or bar of chocolate. Now, looking back on each attempted diet, how long were you able to sustain that diet before the cravings and the hunger got too much? Guess what?! This is not your failing. This is your body simply doing what it is designed to do...survive! This is not a 'willpower' issue! This is a far more deep-rooted problem and one that has been set upon us by today's society of processed foods, promoted snacking and an abundance of sugary, refined foods. The combination of these all play their part in causing a hormone imbalance which ultimately leads to weight gain and makes losing weight so difficult to achieve. The CORRECT advice of WHAT to eat and WHEN to eat is not commonly advertised. Our bodies are controlled entirely by our hormones and here lies the answer we all need to know.

So, referring to this master hormone, Leptin. To put it simply; this hormone controls our desire to eat by communicating with our brain to trigger hunger and then stops us from eating more by communicating with our brain again to trigger feelings of satiety, the feeling of being full-up. Like everything in life however, it is only good while it works and this is the problem; In today's society of sugar, fast food and convenience meals, a hormone imbalance has been created and the Leptin-brain communication doesn't work as it is supposed to. This hormone imbalance causes a Leptin Resistance which affects so many women who are completely unaware that this is what is preventing their weight loss and more than that, is what is causing them to eat more and put weight on.

Leptin is the master hormone that regulates body fat. It is responsible for our energy balance; controlling our calorie intake and expenditure, or more simply, dictating how much we eat and how much energy we burn. Leptin controls how much fat we store in our bodies. Leptin tells the brain how much energy is stored within the body and if more is needed. If these signals to the brain work in the correct manner, the following cycle happens: we eat, leptin controls the expenditure of calories and the storage of body fat, leptin signals to the brain that no more energy is needed and our bodies function efficiently, storing only the body fat that is needed and burning the rest as energy.

Leptin Resistance is a malfunction within this leptin-brain communication and the brain does not receive the message from leptin. It is almost as if the brain's leptin receptors have been switched off. The result being, the brain does not receive the message from leptin signalling that no more energy is needed. When no message is received by the brain, it automatically reverts to survival mode and works to 'call in' more energy in a bid to survive against starvation. The brain does this in two ways: firstly, by sending out cravings. These cravings are what you experience and cannot ignore or fight. It is your brain protecting your body and telling you that you need to eat more, although you already have plenty of energy stored. Secondly, the brain will preserve energy expenditure. It does this by burning fewer calories and operates the body more slowly. This is the lethargic feeling you feel and is often the reason you reach out for that chocolate bar mid-afternoon.

Leptin Resistance is a hormonal defect that is causing so many of us to eat more and exercise less. Once unknown, Leptin Resistance is now fast becoming recognised as the pivotal defect contributing to weight gain and obesity. Many of us now experience Leptin Resistance and it is this that we need to fix within our own bodies in order to lose weight.

Leptin Resistance is a complex issue and can be more apparent in some than it is in others. However, it is becoming commonly recognised that a hormone imbalance caused by overeating and poor diets of refined and sugary foods has caused the Leptin Resistance within us. It is this Leptin Resistance that causes the cravings and overeating that I'm sure you can all relate to; take the evening munchies for example. You are sitting on the sofa, relaxing before going to bed, and there is not a single thing you can do to stop yourself from getting the biscuits out, or diving into your favourite chocolate bar. You know you shouldn't be eating this but you have talked yourself into it. You have fought against it but your mind has put up a good argument, and after all 'there is always tomorrow', right? Night time cravings are in themselves an indication of Leptin Resistance.

Our metabolism is not designed to deal with a constant supply of food and therefore snacking is not the answer to weight loss. It does not maintain the metabolism, it destroys it. It is impossible to eat anything without causing a rise in insulin levels. Once insulin levels rise, so too do leptin levels. The cycle of storing and burning energy is interrupted and the fat burning process is switched off, meaning the energy that was being burned will now be turned to fat and stored instead. So, in a simplified scenario, if for example you have your breakfast at 7am, the leptin hormone will spend the following hours organising the storage and usage of the energy you have just eaten. The energy needed by the body to function will be used and the energy not used to operate the body will be transferred to fat cells and stored. In other words, if this process is left to run its course only the fat needed for the body to survive will be stored and the remainder will be used as energy for the body to function efficiently. The more active you are during this period, the more energy will be used. However, if a snack is consumed between breakfast and lunch, this process has been broken and the fat burning process stopped. The energy that had been consumed at breakfast will be transferred to fat and is then simply stored instead of burned and the body will turn to the newly supplied energy to use instead.

Leptin Resistance can occur for many complex reasons and is a result of a malfunction of the brain's leptin receptor; the receptors have been suppressed by a constant supply of overeating, eating the wrong foods and eating at the wrong time. It is a direct result of an abundance of an unhealthy food supply, and the wrong information promoted about how to lose weight and what diet to follow.

It is a sad fact that the leptin hormone is not more commonly understood, and information on this master hormone is certainly not shared openly with the general public. Instead we are left to float from diet to diet, blissfully unaware that with every diet we try, every snack we munch on and every weight loss short cut we attempt, we are simply creating a stronger

Leptin Resistance. The problem here is that the longer this cycle is left to continue, the weaker the body's metabolism is and ultimately, the harder it becomes to lose weight. In fact, the longer this cycle runs, the more weight is actually gained.

The only way to beat the cycle is to 'fix' the Leptin Resistance. Leptin Resistance can be reversed over time by following some basic principles. L.I.F.E. Fit- The Process takes you through my L.I.F.E. Fit programme, which is a combination of these principles and the results are life changing.

For far too long, far too many magazines and fitness experts have preached that to lose weight is a simple task of 'eat less, exercise more' and whilst this statement is correct, putting this into practice is entirely different. If it really was this easy then we would live in a world of perfectly proportioned, toned individuals. Unfortunately, whilst the principle is correct, there are far more underlying complexities to consider. Not only is it difficult to follow any form of restrictive diet over a period of time when trying to incorporate it into your daily life, once Leptin Resistance is present the cravings for food which are demanded by the brain will always be far stronger than your willpower to not overeat or to make the correct food choices. Now, hopefully you will see that your weight gain is not simply down to self-infliction. Not entirely! Were you aware of what you needed to do to make sure your body is using and storing energy efficiently or were you simply floating from diet to diet in the hope that each one would be the one that worked? Searching the internet each week looking for the newest miracle solution? How are you expected to make the right food choices and exercise effectively when there are so many conflicting diet methods out there? When each new diet programme that hits the headlines turns out to be yet another fad diet that will simply set each of us up to fail? Weight loss is not about cutting out food groups and following some overcomplicated menu plan. It is about fuelling your body correctly and eating with enough time between foods to allow your hormones to do what they are intended to do. It shouldn't be any more complicated than that and any diet that is will soon leave you feeling disillusioned, discouraged and ready to fall hard into your old habits in a disheartened slump. It is this very cycle that we need to stop. Stop following diets, they will harm you in the long term.

L.I.F.E. Fit - The Process will detail each surprisingly simple principle to reverse the Leptin Resistance and balance your leptin levels, meaning your body will function exactly as it is intended to function. The longer L.I.F.E. Fit - The Process is followed, the more efficiently your body will function. The result will not simply be weight loss; you will feel completely in control of your body. You will be completely in control of food and you will feel a sense of empowerment which will show as confidence and energy levels that will surpass your expectations. The result on your body will be leaner, toned and defined muscles, less body fat and a smaller, leaner waistline as your body starts to function exactly as it is intended to do.

The best thing is, you can start L.I.F.E. Fit at any fitness level, at any weight and at any age and the only limit of how far you can take it are the goals you set yourself. Don't tell me the sky is the limit when there are footprints on the moon. Set your goals and believe in yourself.

Now, by reading this far I hope you can see that weight loss is not about eating nothing but cabbage soup or acai berries for 4 weeks. It is a lifestyle and it does need an understanding of what foods are going to benefit your body. This is something you will learn to understand as you follow L.I.F.E. Fit - The Process and will soon become second nature to you. Don't panic, I am not going to tell you to never eat a take-away, or to never pick up chocolate again. L.I.F.E. Fit works in real life and if you are like me real life includes take-away food and the occasional chocolate bar. The Process will give you an understanding of your body, what it needs and how it works; our bodies are under the control of our hormones; the master being leptin. Eat in harmony with leptin and this master hormone will turn your body into a fat burning furnace and all your weight loss efforts will fall into place. You will finally be in control of your body.

So how can my L.I.F.E. Fit programme work for you? By reading this book and following the principles, you will learn what foods your body needs to make it function at its best and more importantly, WHEN you should be eating to allow your hormones the time they need to deal with the energy supply you are providing. This book is an introduction intended to teach you HOW to eat to allow your hormones to function as they need to, allowing them to burn energy and store only the fat that the body needs and nothing else. This book gives you a list of meals that you can pick from every day, making it easy for you to cater for you and your family. Yes, that is right, you get to choose what meals you have rather than being told what meal to have. The meals are broken down into menus for breakfasts, lunches, dinners and desserts plus a selection of snack choices for your children. The recipe for all the meals in each of the menus are also in this book for you, so all you need to do is pick what you want to eat and follow the recipe. Every meal is based on real family favourite meals so can be enjoyed by the whole family. I have included some of my favourite recipes that you can easily prepare and cook with your children; children generally love getting involved in the kitchen and are more likely to eat a meal that they have helped to prepare with you. Okay so the presentation may not be restaurant standard when left to the children to serve but what does that matter when you and your children are getting good, home-cooked, healthy meals? All the ingredients to make the recipes are easily found in any supermarket or health food shop. The recipes are easy to follow and the food is normal, everyday food that you can enjoy with your children. I cook for my family every day and Sean, my 12-year-old son, and my stepsons Kalan and Jesse who are 13 and 17 all eat the same meals that I cook for me and my husband, Dean. You don't need a degree in domestic science to pull a meal together when following L.I.F.E. Fit - The Process. That said, you can get as adventurous with your meals as your domestic abilities allow you to. This book will let you know what foods and ingredients should be avoided, at least within the initial weeks of following L.I.F.E. Fit. This is a progressive programme designed to 'fix' Leptin Resistance. Once your leptin hormone and brain communication is functioning effectively and Leptin Resistance is no longer present, you will be in a better position to be able to eat other foods that should be avoided in the initial weeks. I love chocolate and find it very difficult to say no to a slab of sponge cake. I did however avoid these foods initially to allow my leptin levels to balance and to reverse my Leptin Resistance. Now however, if I want a chocolate bar and fancy a slice of cake, or want to have a family take-away night then I will. I will always bear in mind the principles of my programme and everything I eat will be eaten at a mealtime. Following L.I.F.E. Fit - The Process will not stop you from enjoying 'dirty' food but initially you will need to avoid certain things to allow your body time to rectify the Leptin Resistance and allow your hormones to level. You will learn what to eat and when to eat as you work through this book and the principles will soon become a way of life to you. I know this can often be a scary thought, someone telling you that you are going to learn a 'new way of life', but honestly, it's not that scary. It is not actually a 'new way of life' but more a few simple changes leading to a healthier lifestyle. This book will take you through the principles of my programme and will give you everything you need. You will learn what foods to buy and what to do with them. Try it and see for yourself how simple it really is and how much of a difference to your body it will really make. You won't see a change if you don't make a change and this book is designed to make that change as simple to follow as it can be.

Now on this note I must point out that children's eating habits are and should remain different from that of an adult. A child is still developing physically and mentally and this puts a huge demand on the body's energy requirements. Children need to eat smaller portions at more regular intervals than us adults, so even when you are following the eating patterns of L.I.F.E. Fit and your children are hungry between meals, do not deny them their snacks. All you need to bear in mind is that children's snacks should not be restricted to sweets, chocolates and crisps. Children will love the breakfast, lunch and dinners offered through this book and will enjoy helping you make these and the snacks you give them can also be fun; help them make fruit kebabs for example, or prepare carpet picnics with vegetable sticks and hummus. Children will always ask for sweets, it seems to be unavoidable and as treats of course children should be allowed to enjoy these foods. Sugary snacks however should be avoided as the regular 'go to' snack. Saying no to sweets and biscuits may cause a tantrum from time to time, especially if your children are used to having sweets and biscuits on demand, but it will be far better in their long term to learn to say 'no' to their requests for sweets all the time. This will get easier, especially if you make fruits and vegetables into fun snack time and your children will soon be asking for a satsuma or a banana instead. Fuelling your children with the right foods will have a huge impact on their mental wellbeing, allowing them to focus on tasks for longer, balancing their mood as their own hormones remain unaffected by a sensible sugar intake. You will notice fewer tantrums in younger children by giving them less sugar and teenagers will remain calmer and more focused. Children's nutrition and 'feeding their brain' is a whole other topic and one that I would love to discuss with you but for the time being, all we need to understand is that by eating a balanced diet and taking control of food in your home, you will ultimately benefit your children on many levels too.

The exercises within L.I.F.E. Fit - The Process is a progressive programme, designed to introduce your body to cardio, body resistance and weight training. Regardless of your fitness level, whether you have never exercised before or already go to the gym every day, you can start my exercise programme at your level. You will not be asked to train at weekends, this will be your rest time. Every session will give you a modified, an intermediary and an advanced version of each move. There will always be a way to further modify or to further increase the intensity of every move so that you can slow yourself down to get through or increase your effort as you get stronger. It really is effective training at its best; just 20 minutes working at your best and you are done for the day. All I will ask is that you really do your best at every session. Build a sweat with every session and believe you can complete the 20 minutes and you will be amazed at how quickly your body responds to your efforts and how quickly the results will come.

So, quite simply, L.I.F.E. Fit - The Process explains my L.I.F.E. Fit programme. It is a progressive programme that guides you through every stage of your weight loss and body toning journey, leaving nothing to guess-work. It tells you what meals you can eat, when to eat and gives you recipes to follow so that you can learn at your own pace how to feed your body. It tells you what exercises to do and how to do them, again allowing you to progress as slowly or as quickly as you need. This is simply The Process for weight and fat loss for any age and any fitness level. This book tells you everything you need to get the results that you want without turning your family life upside down or putting extra pressure on you. Every principle throughout L.I.F.E. Fit - The Process really is remarkably simple but amazingly powerful. You will find yourself in control of your body, in control of the food you and your family eat, in control of the wellbeing of your children's health. You will be more confident not only in how you look but more confident that the home you are running is a happy, healthy home with a happy, healthy mum and happy healthy children.

5

FOCUSING ON YOU

making the decision to change

It is one thing reading this book, now you must put your mind in the right place and follow through. Any change you make has to start with your decision to make that change. A decision to change would have started with a reason leading you to that decision. Do you know your reason for wanting to make this change? By following L.I.F.E. Fit - The Process, you absolutely have the potential to make real changes to your body and to the wellbeing of your family, but first you have to look at yourself and start with an honest reflection. Real change starts from within and that is where you will find the strength and determination to keep you going.

The first question I must ask you is...

1. **Have you made the decision to change?**

A) _____

Go on, write your answer down. Remember, this is your book, these are your notes. Be honest with yourself and refer to your answers when you are finding things hard. These will be your motivation buttons to keep you going throughout your journey. The more honest you can be with yourself now, the more motivation these answers will be when you look back at them.

Now the big question....

2. **What is your reason for wanting to make this change?**

A) _____

   _____

   _____

   _____

For some people this answer will be easy, it will be the thoughts that keep you awake at night and haunt you throughout the day. For some of you the answer may be a niggling thought at the back of your mind, reminding you that something in your life needs to change. Either way, you are reading this book for a reason and this is your chance to make the changes. Remember, you need to be honest with yourself!

3. **What do you see when you look at yourself naked in the mirror? Describe how you see your own body.**

A) _____

   _____

   _____

   _____

4. **Do you feel confident about yourself? Explain your answer.**

A) _____

   _____

   _____

   _____

5. **How do you really feel about yourself, how does that make you feel emotionally?**

A) _____
    _____
    _____
    _____

6. **Do you feel confident naked in front of your spouse?**

A) _____

7. **Do you really want to change?**

A) _____

8. **Now look at the food you are offering your children. Being completely honest, are you happy with the food you are giving them?**

A) _____

9. **Do you want your children to benefit physically and mentally from healthy, home-cooked meals prepared by you?**

A) _____

10. **Do you want to be your children's inspiration as they grow up?**

A) _____

11. **What life do you want for you children? Describe how you want them to grow physically. Describe how happy you want them to be. Describe how healthy you want them to be as they grow into young adults and beyond.**

A) _____
_____
_____
_____

12. **Do you believe that if you were to continue with the habits you are currently following at home that you and your children will fully grow to benefit from a healthy, active lifestyle?**

A) _____

13. **How do you want your children to view you? What would you like them to learn from you throughout their childhood? Describe what memories you want your children to take with them into their adulthood**

A) _____
_____

14. **Being honest with yourself, do you believe you and your family are as healthy and active as you could be?**

A) _____

15. **Do you want to be in control of your home, of the lifestyle that you and your family lead?**

A) _____

If you have answered 'yes' to question 1 and you have made the decision to change then there is only one thing left for you to.... Make the change!

So, we have already identified what it is you want to change. Now, to change something successfully requires you to have a vision of what you want the end product to be. In this case, you need a strong vision of what you want to look like and a clear idea of how you want to feel. I have always used visual aids to keep myself motivated. Something that gives me a quick reminder of what I am trying to achieve. There are many social media sites that offer an abundance of motivational pictures. I like to cut these out and have them stuck to walls and cupboards around my house. Things that I may not always look at consciously but they are always in my vision. You can use anything; pictures of you when you were at your most confident, pictures of athletes in motion, pictures of you and your children in the park or on the beach, pictures of that summer dress you are desperate to wear next summer or the bikini you really want to look your best in on your next family holiday. Stick these pictures up around your house. Let them motivate you and inspire you.

Use this space here to write down what you want to achieve by following L.I.F.E. Fit - The Process. Describe how energetic you want to feel throughout each day and how you want your body to look. Set your goals on paper, write down what your ideal weight is and what body fat percentage you want to get to. Write down what dress size you want to be and describe the bikini you want to be able to wear with confidence. Describe how you want to feel in your jeans and detail the shorts you want to feel confident in. Describe how you want to feel as you button up your jeans and how you want your legs to look as you walk in your shorts. Describe the muscle definition you want to see. Describe how healthy you want to be and how energetic you want feel. Describe how healthy you want your children to be. Describe how confident you want your children to be as they grow up. Describe what you want them to grow up into, detail the lifestyle you want for them. Describe the fun you want to have with your children and describe how you want them to be proud of you. Get your pen and write it all down, everything. This is what you will be working for when you are following L.I.F.E. Fit - The Process. And guess what.... this is what you WILL achieve if you follow L.I.F.E. Fit- The Process entirely! Go on.... write down what you and your family **are going to** become!!

_____

_____

_____

_____

_____

_____

_____

_____

_____

_____

_____

_____

_____

_____

_____

_____

6

TIME TO COMMIT

time to plan and prepare

OK, so we are getting the point where I need to start talking less and letting you know what you need to do to start your own journey. I am hoping that you can now see that the age-old advice of simply eating less and exercising more is as much help to you as me handing you a chocolate dumbbell! I wish it was as easy as just eating less and exercising more. Can you imagine if it was that easy? There certainly wouldn't be a whole selection of fitness experts all giving a whole selection of different advice and there would be no confusion about what is to be done. No, it is not that easy and your progress will differ for each of you reading this book, depending on things like age, gender and physical ability. Each of you reading this book will be starting at different points in your health and fitness journey and therefore your journeys will each be different from one another. But that doesn't mean it is impossible and by following L.I.F.E. Fit - The Process, your weight loss journey can be fun and it will certainly be very rewarding. At this point, before I go any further, what I would suggest is that you establish a good support network. Make sure your mum, your sister, your brother, your boyfriend, your husband, your wife, your girlfriend, your best friend...anyone, make sure they are there for you and are ready to help you. This is a process that really does benefit everyone after all. By following my programme, you are going to improve your health, your fitness, your body shape and the health and fitness of your family now and long into the future. As a parent, you need to understand that what your children see you doing, see you eating and see the habits you follow are what they will grow up eating and doing themselves, and what better gift to give your children than the knowledge that living a healthy, fit life is nothing but normal, it's simply what they grew up with.

Before I move on to shopping lists and menus, I want to point something out to you; whilst you might be highly motivated and raring to go at this point, and I do hope you are, there will be times where you are struggling to keep motivated. Times when you have had a week from hell, more bad hair days than hours of sleep and your kitchen cupboards have nothing in them and a trip to the supermarket is a mission in itself. There will be days where even 20 minutes of exercise seems impossible and you feel like you are losing the battle. It is times like this where you will feel pretty low and everything else going on in your life will take priority over what you need to be doing to stay 'on track'

When you are finding things hard and every day seems like a struggle, don't beat yourself up over it. Praise yourself for how far you have come and believe in yourself and all that you are doing. Don't let a bad day or a bad mood or a difficult situation be the thing that beats you! Be strong for yourself and keep going. There will always be little things in everyday life that may present a challenge. I have listed a few common questions and answers here that will hopefully be a helpful quick reference for you to turn to during times like this. The best thing to remember is to prepare in advance and keep things simple.

Q: I can't find the time to exercise. What can I do instead?

A: The truth is, none of us can 'find' the time to exercise. If you have decided that you need to change your body, it is not about 'finding' time but 'making' time. Every training session is just 20 minutes, that's it. If you only have time to train while your children's bath is running…. guess what… that is your work out time! If you have to be somewhere for 9am sharp and you won't get back home until dinner time, get up half an hour earlier or make it the first thing you do when you get home. If you are at home with your children, make it your 20-minute fun session with them. If the only time you have at all during the day is when your children get home from school, then give them your stop watch and ask them to time your intervals, or see if they can compete with you. If you have a husband, wife, boyfriend, girlfriend at home, they can work out with you, encourage you or simply leave you alone for 20 minutes. I know it sounds like a big change to your daily routine but it really doesn't take long before your 20 minutes training becomes a routine in itself. You need to make this change to see a change. It won't be long before your children are asking when you can train because they are looking forward to it. It doesn't matter where you are or what time of day it is, you can be upstairs, downstairs, at your parents, round a friend's house for your children's playdate… literally anywhere. Turn your lounge into a gym, invite your friends round and workout together. You can't beat a workout buddy for motivation. Just remind yourself how good you feel once you have finished your workout and get started. Sometimes, you just need to start before your brain realises what you are doing.

However, all that said if there is a day looming in your diary that will make it impossible to train and there is not a single thing you can do about it or you are feeling so under the weather all you need is a sofa day, then don't train. It is that simple. There is no point beating yourself up over it. The one thing that is important to remember is NOT to fall into the trap of 'I'm not training today so I might as well eat whatever I want, whenever I want' If you cannot train on a particular day, this is the day that you should monitor your food intake more than normal. Whilst the saying 'eat less exercise more' simplifies a complex issue, it is true to say that you need to burn more calories than you eat. Therefore, if you are not training on a particular day then you will be burning fewer calories that day and therefore you need to take in fewer calories. So, if you have a day where missing your training session is unavoidable, then miss it, get on with your day and look forward to training the following day.

Q: I often meet with friends for coffee but they always have cake and biscuits on the table. It is hard to resist eating these with my coffee. How can I stop myself?
A: Firstly, it will only be the initial weeks of L.I.F.E. Fit - The Process where I will ask you to avoid various foods. The longer you follow L.I.F.E. Fit, the more capable your body will be of efficiently coping with foods such as cakes and biscuits. I'm not saying they should be eaten as part of your daily menu but in reality, who can honestly say they are *never* going to eat a slice of cake again? It simply isn't realistic. So, to answer the question, if you know you are going to be in a situation where there will be food that you should initially be avoiding or food available in between your meals, then preparation is important. Plan your meals so that you will not be hungry while you are there. For example, if you are meeting at 1.30pm have your lunch immediately before you go. Remember when I said that your mind plays a key role in your success? It is times like this where you must keep a strong mind. If you are in the initial stages of L.I.F.E. Fit - The Process, you must have made the decision to change. It is times such as this where you must remind yourself of why you want to make that change and what you are aiming to achieve by making the change. Hopefully this reminder will be what it takes to remove the appeal of any cake or biscuit that is in front of you. You

will give in sometimes and that custard cream will get the better of you. Don't beat yourself up over it. If you have eaten it, it's gone. Move on. DON'T let that one biscuit (or cake, or chocolate or large bucket of popcorn or whatever it may be) be the excuse to continue eating throughout the day. That is where the damage will be caused. If you overeat on one occasion or eat something you should initially be avoiding, don't fall into the all too common trap of "I've eaten that now, I may as well carry on today and start again tomorrow" Draw a line there and then. Tomorrow is always too far away to start again.

As I said, the longer you follow L.I.F.E. Fit, the more efficient your body will become and you will be able enjoy the occasional sweet treat or take-away. Eating the foods you enjoy is part of life and to say that you will never eat a particular food again is the first step to failing! By following L.I.F.E. Fit - The Process, as long as you incorporate your treats into a mealtime there is nothing you can't enjoy. That will come in time and by then you will know your body and what it needs.

Q: I simply haven't got the time to prepare fresh meals every day. How can I eat fresh home-cooked meals if I haven't got time to cook the meals?

A: Time is our biggest enemy. We never have enough of it. Unless you are at home all day with nothing else to do then I agree, finding time to prepare nice, fresh meals is hard to come by. I get that. There are a few little tips to help make this easier. These are a few things that I do at home to help me in the kitchen.

1. Supermarkets stock a great range of fresh and frozen pre-chopped vegetables and fruit that can simply be tipped from the bag. These are perfect for freshly cooked meals without the preparation time. Or, get your children involved and ask them to help you chop a selection of vegetables. Give them challenges such as, who can chop the neatest carrot slices, or who can chop the most in 2 minutes... Not only will this give you a stock of prepared vegetables to use, it will get your children engaged in healthy food preparation, which in turn leads on to a natural desire to eat the food they have prepared.

2. When you cook a favourite meal, cook more portions than you need and freeze the rest so that you always have a meal ready to go in the freezer. For example, when you cook a spaghetti bolognaise, cook a big batch of it and tip some into freezer

containers. That way, the next time you want that meal, all you need to do is cook the spaghetti and re-heat the bolognaise. Remember, this can not only be done if you are cooking with meat that has not previously been frozen.

3. Plan your meals in advance so that you can take out of the freezer anything that you will need for the following day. Come meal time, they will be as quick to cook as any processed food.

4. Keep your kitchen well stocked. When you are running low on ingredients, grab more! Being prepared and having the right food choices available is key to making good food choices each day. Always have a healthy 'go to' ingredient in your cupboards to use on the days when you have nothing else left in the house. I always keep tins of tuna and packets of quick cook basmati rice in my cupboard and chicken in my freezer as my emergency 'go to' food.

5. Throw away any processed foods that are in your kitchen and do not buy any more. Don't even look at them when you go shopping. If it's not in your house, you can't eat it.

6. Keep your meal choices simple. A healthy meal does not have to be a complicated meal. We're not trying to be master chefs here.

The recipes that I have included in this book are simple, quick to prepare and easy to cook. I have to prepare meals quickly at home, I haven't got hours to spend in the kitchen; I have a job to do, a house to run and children to enjoy. I have included the recipes that I cook at home on a regular basis. If you have the right ingredients in your kitchen, especially if they are already chopped for you, then cooking a healthy home cooked meal is as quick as heating through a processed meal. Remember, the more processed something is, the more harm it will do to your body and your children's overall health.

7

THE PRINCIPLES

trust The Process

These are the principles of my L.I.F.E. Fit programme and are the remarkably simple steps of The Process; it is important that you understand each of the principles so that you can appreciate the importance of following them. L.I.F.E. Fit - The Process will only work for you if you follow these principles entirely. It is important to be strict with yourself on these principles because they are the foundation of fat burning success. By following these principles, you will be reversing Leptin Resistance by balancing your hormones, which will in turn fix and increase your metabolism which will drop your body weight. Stick to these principles and you too will unlock the answer to weight control and fat loss without the dieting. I wish I could fast forward you a few weeks into the future so that you could see and feel the difference in your body and mind. Read these principles, learn them, live by them and TRUST THE PROCESS!

WHAT YOU MUST DO

- Eat breakfast within one hour of waking up
- Eat three meals a day and do not snack in between
- Allow five hours between each meal
- Control portion size
- Allow three hours after dinner before going to bed

EAT BREAKFAST WITHIN ONE HOUR OF WAKING UP

Breakfast is needed to fuel your body after the over-night fasting period. Your body works hard overnight while you sleep and upon waking needs a new source of energy to draw from. Without a breakfast to re-fuel the body, your metabolism will run slower in an effort to preserve energy, meaning you will be burning fewer calories overall. Without a breakfast to sustain you in the morning you will be left feeling hungrier late morning leading up to lunchtime and will me more likely to make poor food choices and over-eat at lunch. I understand that breakfast often needs to be quick to prepare as there is very little time in the morning when you have school runs, work commutes, maybe a baby to cater for or a toddler to entertain. The breakfast menu gives you options ranging from quick and easy weekday breakfast as well as weekend breakfasts when you may have more time to sit and enjoy breakfast more leisurely.

EAT THREE MEALS A DAY AND DO NOT SNACK IN BETWEEN

Our metabolism is not capable of dealing with a constant supply of food. Food is simply an energy source for our bodies. If a surplus of energy is supplied to our bodies, the body has no option but to store the extra supply and it can only do this by transferring it into fat cells. If you eat a fresh supply of energy before your body has used the previous supply, your body will simply store it as body fat. Allowing your body to use the energy supplied by each meal without interruption will see your body using the energy it needs and storing only the essential fats required for normal body function.

It is important to remember that children's and teenagers' bodies and brains are still developing and are doing so at a remarkable rate, and therefore this no snacking rule does NOT apply to them. Children and teenagers will use the energy supply from each meal far quicker than adults and they do need a snack between meals to sustain their development. I have included a snacks and sides menu so that you can pick healthy snacks to give your children so they can continue to enjoy the snacks they need and you can have peace of mind knowing that they are eating enough without overdoing the sugar intake.

ALLOW FIVE HOURS BETWEEN EACH MEAL

This is the fat burning process. Once a meal is eaten, the adult body will use this time to 'organise' the energy supply from that meal, transferring what is needed by the body into essential fats and using the rest to function. The more active you are during this time, the more energy your body will use from the meal. Your body will continue to use the available energy from the meal to get your body through the activities you are asking of it, drawing from stored fat cells if all the energy supply from the meal is used up. Alternatively, if your next meal is eaten within this time, the body will have a new energy supply to use and will either stop drawing from stored body fat or, if it was still using available energy from the first meal, will now transfer this into fat cells and store it as body fat instead. Allowing the five hours to pass between each meal is fundamental in reversing Leptin Resistance and balancing your hormones. The longer you feed your body in this way, the more efficient your body becomes at burning body fat.

CONTROL PORTION SIZE

Every meal you have should be sufficient to see you through the five hours to your next meal. As the five hours pass, you should be hungry and ready to eat your next meal, but not so hungry that you are climbing in your kitchen cupboards and ready to eat your children. It is important then to think about what you eat for each meal, remembering that fresh foods that provide your body with essential macronutrients will sustain your appetite far more than processed, convenience foods. Macronutrients are simply complex carbohydrates, protein and good fats. Every meal should provide you with a source of each of the three macronutrients. These meals will fill you up quicker therefore preventing you from eating portions that are too big and will also leave you feeling fuller for longer, preventing you from getting too hungry between meals.

The correct portion size varies from person to person depending on various things such as size, age and activity levels. Many of us do not have an 'off' signal when we eat, causing us to eat everything on our plate. If you have served up a portion that is too large, the chances are you will eat it all even if you have stopped feeling hungry. So how do you know what the correct portion size is for you? The easiest guide is to use your hand. Loose foods such as vegetables, rice or pasta should be measured in the palm of your hand; if you can hold it in your hand then you can eat it. An item of food such as chicken breast or potato should be no bigger than your fist.

When you have finished your meal, remember it can take about twenty minutes before you feel full up. If you feel hungry straight after your meal, allow yourself twenty minutes before you re-fill your plate with a second helping. If after the twenty minutes you are genuinely hungry, have a dessert from the desert menu.

Meal-times should be savoured. A time when you can sit at your dinner table with your family and talk about your day. Or if your family routine doesn't allow for you to all eat together then use your mealtimes to enjoy a moment of calm. Don't try to rush a meal, enjoy it. Were you always being told to eat slower when you were younger? Perhaps it's something you need to say to your own children now? It's a good piece of advice! By eating slowly, you are allowing your body the time to recognise when it has had enough to eat and to pass the signal to your brain telling you when you are full. But for you to fully appreciate the food you are eating and to allow your brain to recognise the messages of being full up it is important to stop whatever you are doing at each mealtime. Sit down to eat and enjoy every mouthful. Your brain can not register that you are full up if you are concentrating on the TV, reading a book or scrolling through a smartphone or tablet. Stop, enjoy your food then carry on with the other stuff.

One thing I do to stop myself from eating too fast is to eat the food from my fork but then not organise the next forkful until I have chewed and swallowed. Once I have swallowed a mouthful, I will then look at my plate and put more food on my fork. If you are planning your next mouthful while chewing you will be thinking more about what is on your fork rather than what is in your mouth. By enjoying every mouthful before placing more on your fork will naturally slow down your eating.

As a mum, I fully appreciate just how fussy our children can be when it comes to the food they eat. Don't despair if your children always turn their nose up at the food you give them. Keep persevering and try to keep calm about it. Children will find their own way and if you keep offering the good stuff, it will eventually start to get eaten. It is important to not overload their plates because many children can find a full plate quite overwhelming. Their meals should be very much smaller than that of an adult and if your child states that they are full up before their plate is empty it is important to accept this. Allow them to leave food on their plate if they are full. When they are next hungry they will tell you and you can decide on what to give them at that point. Forcing a child to finish a meal just because the food is on their plate is doing nothing more than reinforcing the very habit we are trying to break ourselves. Just because it is on the plate, it doesn't mean you must eat it. Listen to your body and allow your children to do the same.

ALLOW THREE HOURS AFTER DINNER BEFORE GOING TO BED

Your body is very busy when you are asleep, repairing and restoring itself which uses a lot of energy. This means your body still uses energy even when you are sleeping. If you lay your yourself down to sleep for the night too soon after eating, your body will use the energy supply from your dinner to generate its repairing process, rather than drawing the required energy from stored body fat. To make matters worse, your body will go on to store any energy it doesn't use as more body fat and as a result you would have increased your body fat overnight rather than using it.

If you allow time for your body to use the energy from your dinner before going to sleep, your body will then be forced to draw the energy needed for the repair process from stored fat cells, transferring these back into energy instead.

Many people confuse this time needed before going to bed by saying that food should not be eaten after a certain time in the evening. Think about that statement! How does your body know what time it is?! Your body does not know how to tell the time. Your body doesn't know if you eat your dinner at 5PM or 10PM and it really doesn't matter either way, as long as you allow your body the time it needs to use the energy from that meal before laying your body down to sleep.

<u>HELPFUL TIPS</u>

- Choose meals that will deliver the required macronutrients to your body. You need complex carbohydrates, protein and good fats in each meal
- Processed foods will not give your body what it needs
- Processed foods will not be sufficient to sustain you for five hours
- Eat slowly
- Stop eating when you are full, never continue to eat until you are 'stuffed'
- Try to reduce your caffeine intake. Green tea makes a great replacement. If you can't get through the day without your caffeine, try drinking it black. If you can't drink it black use a milk alternative instead of milk, such as almond milk or soya milk
- Complete your work out sessions
- Drink water, drink water, drink water! You need to be drinking at least 2 litres of water every day, plus whatever you drink during your work out.

To make each day easier it is important to stay focused in the evening. As you continue to eat the right foods at the right time and in the correct portions, the cravings will start to diminish. Soon enough you will realise that you do not need the extra snacks between each meal, nor do you want them.

The important thing to remember is that you are not being told that you should never eat anything with sugar in it again or that you can never order a take-away pizza again. If you were to tell yourself you were never again going to eat a slice of cake, or never going to indulge in your favourite biscuits or that you can never enjoy a meal out with friends or family you will be setting yourself up for a fall. Once you have given your body the chance for the Leptin Resistance to be 'fixed' then your body will be in a better position to deal with 'treats' and it is not necessary to avoid them completely. Everything in moderation after all. What you need to remember is to always incorporate your 'treats' into a mealtime. If you want a bar of chocolate, have it with your lunch. If you want a croissant, have it with breakfast. If you are planning on a slice of cake, make it your dessert. It would take a highly-disciplined person to never eat these foods and it is highly unfair of any FAD diet to make you feel guilty about having these indulgencies from time to time. I enjoy these foods as much as anyone. That doesn't mean I eat them every day and when I do, I always incorporate them into one of my meals.

DRINK WATER

I've said it before and I will say it again. Drink water. This can't be emphasised enough. When you wake up in the morning, drink one pint of cold water before you do anything else. Then fill up a 2-litre bottle of water and drink from this throughout the day. Make sure this bottle is empty before you go to bed. The water you drink while you are working out is to be in addition to your 2-litre bottle. Drink water!

Initially you will find yourself visiting the bathroom more frequently, quite a lot more to be honest. This is good. It shows that your body is flushing unwanted toxins from your body, which in turn will help the weight loss process.

QUICK REFERENCE

So, to recap, the principles to live by are simply;

1. EAT BREAKFAST WITHIN ONE HOUR OF WAKING UP

2. EAT THREE MEALS A DAY AND DO NOT SNACK IN BETWEEN

3. ALLOW FIVE HOURS BETWEEN EACH MEAL

4. CONTROL PORTION SIZE

5. ALLOW THREE HOURS AFTER DINNER BEFORE GOING TO BED

6. FOLLOW THE EXERCISE PROGRAMME

FOODS TO AVOID

In terms of what you can eat, remember, you are not following a FAD. As I have said before, you will not be asked to remove entire food groups from your diet. In fact, nothing is off limits. What you are asked to do is to be mindful about what you do eat. Enjoy 'treats' in moderation and as part of a meal, remember your goals and enjoy the journey.

To help balance your hormones and re-ignite your metabolism, I am going to ask you to avoid two things completely throughout the first two weeks and to enjoy in moderation thereafter.

1. REFINED SUGAR

Including foods and drink that contain refined sugar (yes, that does include alcohol)

Refined sugar has no nutritional benefit and does your body harm. By removing this one item from your diet will have a dramatic and positive impact on your weight loss.

Sugar is addictive. The more you have the more your body will crave. In reverse, the less you have, the less your body will crave.

After the two-week period, you can have items containing refined IN MODERATION, ideally not daily and only as part of a meal.

2. WHITE STARCH

Such as white bread, white pasta, white rice, crackers and savoury pastries

These foods are simple carbohydrates, which your body doesn't need and are not to be confused with complex carbohydrates. Your body will use simple carbohydrates much in the same way as refined sugar. While you may get a quick burst of energy from them, this is only because they have spiked your insulin levels, in the same way refined sugar does and an energy slump will follow. Any nutritional values in these foods have been stripped in the processing method and therefore will not benefit your health or help your weight loss.

After the two-week period, much in the same way as refined sugar, you can have simple carbohydrates if you wanted to but do so knowing that your appetite will not be satisfied for five hours, your nutritional values will not have been met and your weight loss attempts will be hampered.

REMEMBER! Processed foods and convenience foods will generally contain sugar and white flour, meaning they fall within 1 and 2 above. Two weeks may not sound like a long time but there will be times, especially in the evenings where you will find this hard. Be strong and don't allow yourself to give in to the cravings. They will be strong and will try to beat you. Keep reminding yourself why you are doing this and keep telling yourself it is only for two weeks. You will feel so much better for it and your weight loss journey will be easier for it.

BE GLUTEN AWARE and BE AWARE OF GLUTEN FREE PRODUCTS

Many people choose to avoid gluten even if they are not Celiac. Although you will not be asked to avoid gluten, I would like you to be aware of how you feel when you eat foods that contain gluten. If you feel bloated and lethargic after eating foods that contain gluten, then you may benefit from avoiding these foods. Gluten is often added to many foods such as sausages, pasta sauces, soups, frozen convenience foods and is found in wheat, barley and rye.

That said, if you do decide that you are happier reducing your gluten intake, or even avoiding it altogether, it is very important to remember that 'gluten free' does not mean 'sugar free' Don't be tricked into believing that a food product instantly becomes healthy simply by being gluten free. In the contrary, many gluten free products such as bread, cakes, muffins or sauces contain more sugar than their gluten counterpart. If you decide that you genuinely feel better by not eating foods that contain gluten, make your own gluten free products rather than relying on shop-bought products.

So now you know what you need to do. You have everything you need within the pages of this book to achieve your goals. It is down to you now. You are the only person who can make this happen for you. Remember you always have this book to refer to for guidance whenever you need to. When you feel your motivation wobbling and you forget why you started this journey, refer to your notes. Don't give up on yourself.

This is all you need to do to lose weight, burn body fat and lead a fit and healthy lifestyle for your whole family. There is no measuring, no counting, no impossible restrictions, no complicated routine to live by, just some simple principles to follow that will fit seamlessly into even the busiest of routines. Your children will see you living a healthy life without the imbalanced hormone induced mood swings, the grumbles or complaints, the low energy levels or the meal restrictions. Instead, they will see you enjoying the meals, having fun with physical activity and enjoying 'treats' without over indulging or feeling guilty. This will all lead to you teaching them, through example, what a healthy, fit life is. Something they will grow up with and go on to live themselves as adults.

8

LEARNED BEHAVIOUR

our children pick up on more than we realise

As a parent, you have more power over your children's opinions, beliefs, learned behaviour and overall psychology than anything else in your life; so what are you subconsciously teaching your children with your own behaviours towards food and exercise? Are your behaviours towards your own weight battles unintentionally leading your children towards a poor body image or eating disorder?

Children learn a lot from their parents' behaviour and listen to what we say a lot more than we realise. Little comments that we parent's innocently make can have devastating and long lasting effects on our children. How many times have you innocently said "I can't eat that, I'll get fat" or "You need to lose that tummy or you won't fit your school uniform next term" or "Look at that little girl/boy in your class, isn't he/she thin/fat" maybe you have fallen foul to meal skipping before, saying "I'm not eating dinner today, I'm trying to lose weight for our holiday" These are all comments that children can easily hear us parents say pretty much daily and could be the start of a slippery slope towards growing up with a poor body image themselves. Our comments and behaviours could be the start of a developing low-self-esteem, which is something no parent wishes for their children.

It is important to remember that your children are witness to every new fad diet you try ready for your next holiday. Every sad or bad mood you experience yourself about losing weight. They see you try all the extreme measures to lose your belly fat and they hear you every time you compare yourself with the mums at the school gate or with the models and celebrities on the pages of the magazines you leave on your coffee table. Our children are under immense pressure in today's society to be 'body perfect' (whatever that is) and children can often fall foul to this pressure, leading to depression, low self-esteem and a poor body image that in growing cases, can lead to eating disorders. This affliction is not exclusive to girls. Boys are under just as much pressure in today's world to be 'body perfect'

On the other end of the spectrum, your children will see you as you eat your way through every packet of biscuits whilst watching your favourite TV programme and will innocently copy you as you eat crisps with every lunch followed by a chocolate bar in between meals. As a child, if this is what they see their parents doing daily, they will naturally grow up following the same habits themselves because it is what they would have learned. This will only lead to your children hiding their bodies behind baggy clothes and experiencing the same negative body images and low self-esteem about their weight as you experience yourself.

As parents, we need to keep our children from becoming ill through malnutrition from under- eating or overweight from over-eating and the only way we can do that is by leading a balanced, healthy lifestyle ourselves without extreme diets or binge eating. We must lead by example to give our children the best possible chance of growing into healthy, fit and balanced adults themselves.

Unfortunately, the only example of 'body perfect' our children are exposed to and are pressured to live up to are the images of their pop idols and the images in the magazines they read and see on music videos.

Our children learn from their parents before going off to school at which point we can't stop these external influences swarming them. They need their parents to lay a strong positive body image before they are released into the world of school and they need their parents to maintain this positivity towards food and body image throughout their school life. As parents, we can only do that by the behaviours we demonstrate ourselves. To be positive about our own bodies, to be seen to enjoy the foods we eat and share with our family, to be seen to enjoy physical activity and to make this a regular part of family life. As a parent, we cannot be seen to be constantly over-eating the wrong foods, and we cannot be seen to be constantly obsessing over our own weight. Not only does this do ourselves damage and cause us low self-esteem but the damage this can potentially have on our children can be devastating and long-lasting.

By following L.I.F.E. Fit - The Process, the two extremes of over-eating and under-exercising or under-eating and obsessing about diets and exercise are removed. Instead you have nothing but a balanced, healthy lifestyle. Your children will be witness to healthy routines, nutritious and delicious foods and fun, effective physical activity. They will see you happy and confident with your body and with food and will grow up with a stronger positive attitude themselves, ready to pass the same routines to their own children, in time.

9

TIME FOR ACTION

don't be scared – you've got this

Now go into your kitchen and clear out all the processed food. Throw it away, give what you can to your local food bank, do whatever you need to do to get it out of your house. If you haven't got it, you can't eat it. If you have a cupboard where you keep your children's sweets or biscuits, firstly, ask yourself if you want them to have quite so many sugary treats in the house, then ask yourself if you are keeping them for your children, or for you?!
What you do keep for your children for their treats or pack lunches, put in a cupboard away from your food. This would be a good place to keep your motivational pictures and notes as prevention in case you are drawn to this cupboard (and I am sure you will be in the early days).

Once you have cleared your kitchen, it is time to put your mind in the right place. Do not concentrate on the foods you shouldn't be eating. Concentrate on all the foods you should be eating. There are many delicious foods to be enjoyed and you and your family will love them. Don't think for a second you are going to be depriving yourself of food. If anything, you will discover so many foods and meals. Be excited, not daunted. This book will not steer you wrong. Take a flick through the recipes in this book and start getting excited. This is the start of your weight loss journey and a new healthy life for you and your children that will take you all long into your future.

SHOPPING LIST

Here is a shopping list of groceries that you should keep stocked in your kitchen. By having these ingredients, you will be able to follow each of the recipes within this book and will be well on your way to losing weight, toning your body and best of all, being able to provide your children with healthy family meals that they will love and grow healthy from. Meals you can all sit down and enjoy together

PROTEIN

Free-range eggs	Quorn mince	Lentils	Fish – salmon, cod, tuna, seabass
Quorn 'chicken'	Fage Total Greek Yoghurt NOT Greek 'style'	Lean red meat	Cottage cheese (full fat)
Quinoa	Free range chicken	Lean steak mince	Oats
Chia seeds	Turkey mince	Feta cheese (full fat)	Tofu
Spanish Chorizo	Peanut Butter	Mixed Nuts	

CARBOHYDRATES (The complex ones)

VEGETABLES	Garlic	Kale	Spinach
Cabbage	Peas	Carrots	Broccoli
Lettuce (all varieties)	Cauliflower	Courgettes	Onions (red & white)
Bell peppers	Celery	FRUITS	Strawberries
Blueberries	Apples	Tomatoes	Pineapple
Raspberries	Oranges	Bananas	Kiwi fruit
Oranges	Satsumas & clementine	Mangoes	Apricot
brown basmati rice or basmati rice	Brown rice pasta spaghetti & penne	Potatoes White & sweet	

FATS

Avocados	Raw Nuts	100% Organic coconut oil	Olive oil
Coconut milk	Olives	Dark Chocolate (no less than 70% cocoa)	Nut butters
Mozzarella	Haloumi (Or Tofu alternative)		

EXTRAS

Basil (fresh or dried)	Oregano (fresh or dried)	Thyme (fresh or dried)	Chives (fresh or dried)
Cayenne pepper	Chilli powder	Paprika	Black pepper
Garlic puree	Chillies	Green tea	Almond milk (or milk alternative of your choice)
Honey	Passata	Tomato puree	Raw Cacao
Dates	Sultanas & dried fruits	Cinnamon	Maple Syrup

MENUS

I have provided menus for breakfast, lunch, dinner, dessert as well as snacks and sides, all of which you can choose your meals from until you build your confidence with food in terms of what to have and what to do with it. While you are getting used to fresh ingredients and learning what delicious meals you can create, I am going to ask you to pick each of your meals from the menus and use the recipe to create a lovely nutritious family meal. There is enough variety here to make sure you don't get bored and each of the meals are easy to prepare and cook. There is a recipe for each of the meals in the menus for you to refer to as your confidence grows. Every meal is an everyday family favourite that you and your children can enjoy together. No more preparing your own meals separately from your families and cooking several different meals each dinner time – who needs that hassle?!

I am not going to tell you what breakfast, lunch and dinner you are to eat every day for the next 12 weeks, because realistically, that would be very hard to stick to; You may be starting my programme in the summer months so my telling you to eat a chicken hotpot on Tuesday of week 3, for example would be silly.

Instead, each of the meals on the menus are all healthy, nutritious, balanced meals that will fuel your body with the energy it needs and will provide you with the nutrients and calories your body will need to grow strong and burn fat effectively. What's more, each meal listed will also provide the nutrients your children need to allow their bodies and brains to develop healthily and efficiently, allowing them to focus and grow as they should.

Simply select your favourite option for each meal for you and your family each day.

BREAKFAST MENU

Mornings are often busy and rushed so a breakfast that takes minutes to prepare is important. Here are some quick and easy breakfasts for the weekday rush together with a variety of breakfasts to enjoy on the slower Sunday mornings.

- ✓ Scrambled piggy egg
- ✓ 3 Egg, Feta & spinach omelette
- ✓ Chocolate and banana overnight oats
- ✓ Apple and cinnamon overnight oats
- ✓ Bacon bombs
- ✓ Egg and ham baked muffins
- ✓ Chocolate Pancakes
- ✓ Coconutty Pancakes
- ✓ Chocolate orange breakfast cake
- ✓ Apple and cinnamon breakfast cake
- ✓ Smashed avocado bagel with poached egg
- ✓ Breakfast Smoothie

LUNCH MENU

Lunch for some of you will mean planning what to have at home for you and your children. For others, you have to consider what you can prepare for yourself to take to work and for some of you, you also have to consider school lunches. I have incorporated lunch ideas for each of these routines. Any of the egg, bagel or toast choices from the breakfast menu are also great options for lunch. That said, of you had a bagel or toast for breakfast, it is best to choose something else for your lunch.

- ✓ Greek salad
- ✓ Chorizo & red pepper frittata
- ✓ Butternut squash soup
- ✓ Tuna salad
- ✓ French spinach toast with poached egg
- ✓ Stuffed mushrooms with rocket salad
- ✓ Greek chicken pitta pockets
- ✓ One-bowl mixed leaf beetroot salad with feta, ham & egg

DINNER MENU

Dinner is my favourite meal of the day because it is when we all get to sit down as a family. These meals are simple and quick to prepare making them ideal for the busy mid-week dinner and are a great opportunity to get your children involved in cooking.

- ✓ Chilli con carne Y Chilli sin carne
- ✓ Chicken Thai green curry
- ✓ Meatballs and spaghetti
- ✓ Chilli Penne with spinach and Feta
- ✓ Chicken korma
- ✓ Simple Kedgeree
- ✓ Beef Stroganoff
- ✓ Chargrilled chicken with broccoli and Haloumi stack
- ✓ Chicken Cordon Bleu
- ✓ Chicken nuggets
- ✓ Fish fingers
- ✓ Chilli beef stuffed bell peppers
- ✓ Fake-A-Way Pizza
- ✓ Baked cod fillet with Mediterranean roasted vegetables & baked eggs

DESSERT MENU

We all love a dessert and there is no reason to deprive yourself of this pleasure when you are losing weight and burning body fat. On the contrary, the ingredients within these mouth-watering dessert options will provide your body with much needed nutrients. These desserts will change the way you see sweet food with absolutely NO refined sugar used in any of them. Perfect for your waistline and a great platform for a healthy upbringing for your children.

- ✓ Greek volcano
- ✓ Chocolate and walnut brownie
- ✓ Millionaires shortbread
- ✓ 60 second vanilla cake
- ✓ Vanilla nice-cream
- ✓ Kiwi ice-cream
- ✓ Chocolate muffins
- ✓ Strawberry cheesecake balls

CHILDREN'S SNACKS & SIDES MENU

A child's brain develops at a phenomenal rate, creating rapid cognitive, emotional, linguistic and motor developments. As a mum, you have the natural instincts to nourish your child's growing brain through cuddling, cradling, playing, reading, talking to them and singing and all of these things stimulate our children's brain growth and emotional development. However, it is equally as important to nurture your child with healthy food.

The brain requires two major fuel supplies to function properly: oxygen, which is provided by breathing, and glucose (sugar – the natural kind), which is delivered to the brain after the food eaten has been converted to energy.

So, when you are feeding your children, you are not only supporting their growing bodies, you are literally feeding their brain. By providing your children with the correct nutrients through food, what you are actually doing is helping their brain to develop and grow, enabling your child to think more clearly, stay focused and be able to concentrate for longer, be more alert and energetic and deal with stressful situations better. This is all imperative throughout infancy when the brain is growing as the child develops, and into childhood and teenage years when your child is expected to perform throughout their school life and deal with their ever-changing hormones.

So, what are you supposed to give your children to eat to ensure that you are giving their brain everything it needs? Well, in a nutshell it is the same as you would give yourself to be healthy. The snacks and sides menu is intended to give you some ideas for snacks for your children as well as things you may like to incorporate into one of your meals.

- ✓ Wholemeal Loaf
- ✓ Gluten and wheat free loaf
- ✓ Strawberry & coconut jam
- ✓ Tzatziki
- ✓ Granola bars
- ✓ Beetroot salad
- ✓ Lentil pate
- ✓ Oven chips

RECIPES

These recipes are not designed to be an exhaustive list of only the meals you can eat, but rather to give you inspiration and guidance about the sort of foods and meals you can and should be eating. It is time to stop looking at food as an enemy. Your body needs the nutrients delivered by eating the right type of food and the right type of food includes more than most people realise. Enjoy your food and have fun experimenting with recipes. Use these recipes while you gain confidence in your own judgement about what to eat.

BREAKFAST

SCRAMBLED PIGGY EGG

WHAT YOU NEED

Small knob of unsalted butter
(or soya based butter)

Three free range eggs

One sliced good quality ham
(cut into strips)

Chives (fresh or dried)

THE FUN PART

Melt butter in a frying pan

Break the eggs straight into the pan

Stir the eggs constantly, ensuring the yolks are broken

While the eggs are still 'wet' add the ham and chives and continue to stir until eggs are set

serve on 2 slices of wholemeal toast

THREE EGG, FETA & SPINACH OMMELETTE

WHAT YOU NEED

Three free range eggs (whisked)

100g Arla Apetina Classic feta cheese
(or dairy free salad cheese)

1 handful of baby spinach

Extra Virgin Olive Oil

THE FUN PART

Heat a little Olive Oil into a frying pan

Pour the eggs into the pan, tipping the pan
to pour the mixture evenly

Add the spinach evenly over the egg

Crumble the Feta over the spinach

Lift the pan slightly off the heat and move in a
circular motion to avoid the omelette from
sticking

As soon as the egg is set, slide the omelette out
onto a plate and serve

CHOCOLATE AND BANANA OVERNIGHT OATS

(This is to be prepared the night before for a ready to grab breakfast the following morning)

WHAT YOU NEED

40 grams wholegrain porridge oats
(gluten free optional)

300ml Almond milk
(or any milk alternative of your choice)
1 Banana (sliced)

1 dessert spoon of cacao powder
or 1 scoop chocolate protein powder*

1 teaspoon cinnamon

THE FUN PART

Pour the oats into a cereal bowl

Pour the almond milk over the oats and mix
the milk level should be just above the oats

Add the cacao powder (or protein powder) and
the cinnamon and stir well to mix

Arrange the banana slices over the top

Cover with kitchen foil and place in the fridge
overnight, ready for breakfast

If you are making these for children under 16 years old, DO NOT use protein powder

APPLE AND CINNAMON OVERNIGHT OATS

(This is to be prepared the night before for a ready to grab breakfast the following morning)

WHAT YOU NEED

40 grams wholegrain porridge oats
(gluten free optional)

300ml Almond milk
(or milk alternative of your choice)

1 small chopped apple

1 teaspoon Cinnamon

Small handful sultanas

THE FUN PART

Pour the oats into a cereal bowl

Pour the almond milk over the and mix
the milk level should be just above the oats

Add the chopped apple, sultanas and cinnamon
to the oats and stir to mix

Cover with kitchen foil and place in the fridge
overnight, ready for breakfast

BACON BOMBS
(Makes 12 'bombs')
Suggested serving is 2 'bombs' per person)

WHAT YOU NEED

12 rashers bacon

4 free range eggs (whisked)

2 white mushrooms, cut into thin slices

THE FUN PART

Using a muffin tray, line each muffin hole with a
rasher of bacon, ensuring the hole is fully lined
with the bacon

Pour the egg to the top of each muffin hole

Share the mushroom slices between batches

Place in the middle of a pre-heated oven,
gas mark 6, for 20 minutes, or until eggs are set
and the bacon is cooked thoroughly

Serve on wholemeal or gluten free bagel

EGG AND HAM BAKED MUFFINS

WHAT YOU NEED

4 free range eggs (whisked)

2 slices quality ham (cut in strips)

1 dessert spoon Fage Total Greek yoghurt
(or dairy free alternative)

1 teaspoon dried chives

THE FUN PART

Line a muffin tin with muffin cases

Place yoghurt into a bowl and stir in the eggs,
mixing until a creamy consistency is formed

Add the ham into the egg and yoghurt mix

Stir in the chives and mix

Pour the egg mixture into the muffin cases,
filling each one to the top

Place in the middle of a pre-heated oven, gas
mark 6 for 20 minutes or until the egg mix is set

CHOCOLATE PANCAKES
Makes 4 pancakes – 1 serving

WHAT YOU NEED

1 Mashed banana

1 egg (whisked)

1 desert spoon raw cacao powder
or scoop of chocolate protein powder*

Virgin coconut oil

THE FUN PART

Mix all the ingredients together, ensuring all
lumps have gone

Heat the coconut oil in a frying plan

Pour half a ladle of mixture per pancake into
the pan to form pancake rounds

Leave until small bubbles form on top of the
pancake mixture

Flip the pancakes over and leave for a further 1
minute

Stack the pancakes onto a plate

Serve with Fage Total Greek Yoghurt and sliced strawberries
or dairy free plant or soya based yoghurt alternative

If making for children under 16 years old, DO NOT use protein powder

COCONUTTY PANCAKES
Makes 4 pancakes – 1 serving

WHAT YOU NEED

300ml almond milk
(or milk alternative of your choice)

480 grams coconut flour

2 free range eggs

2 rashers bacon

Maple syrup (to serve)

Coconut oil

THE FUN PART

Whisk the flour, milk and eggs together until a stiff, creamy texture is formed

Grill the bacon and place to one side

Heat the coconut oil in a frying pan

Pour half a ladle of mixture per pancake into the pan to form pancake rounds

Leave until small bubbles form on top of the pancakes

Flip the pancakes over and leave for a further 1 minute

Stack the pancakes onto your plate, placing the bacon in between the stacks

Drizzle the stack with maple syrup

CHOCOLATE ORANGE BREAKFAST CAKE

WHAT YOU NEED

40 grams wholegrain porridge oats
(gluten free optional)

1 free range egg (whisked)

1 banana

Juice of one orange

1 teaspoon raw cacao powder
or 1 scoop of chocolate protein shake*

THE FUN PART

Mash the bananas in a cereal bowl until all lumps are removed

Pour the egg into the banana and mix well

Stir the porridge into the egg and banana mix and stir well

Add the cacao powder (or protein powder) to

Stir in the orange juice and mix well until a smooth consistency is formed

Cook in a microwave for 3 minutes or until a fork comes out clean

Serve with a drizzle of honey and orange segments

If making for children under 16 years old, DO NOT use protein powder

APPLE & CINNAMON BREAKFAST CAKE

WHAT YOU NEED

40 grams wholegrain porridge oats
(gluten free optional)

1 free range egg (whisked)

1 banana

1 small apple
(chopped into small cubes)

Small handful of sultanas

1 teaspoon of cinnamon

1 teaspoon of Maple syrup

THE FUN PART

Mash in a cereal, mash the banana until smooth

Pour the egg into the bowl with the banana and
stir to mix well

Stir the porridge oats into the egg and banana
and stir until combined

Add the chopped apple, sultanas, cinnamon and
maple syrup and stir until smooth

Cook in a microwave for 3 minutes or until a
fork comes out clean

Serve with a spoonful of Fage Total Greek yoghurt & chopped hazelnuts
or dairy free plant or soya based yoghurt alternative

SMASHED AVACADO BAGEL WITH POACHED EGG

WHAT YOU NEED

1 wholemeal bagel
(or gluten free bagel)

½ AVACADO

2 free range eggs

Black pepper (to season)

THE FUN PART

Mash the avocado until smooth

Season the avocado with black pepper

Slice the bagel in half and toast on both sides

While the bagel is toasting, crack the eggs into a
deep pan of boiling water and leave for
3 minutes (ensure eggs are cooked) before
removing from water (you can use soft boiled
eggs if preferred)

Spread the avocado evenly on both sides of the
bagel

Scoop the eggs out of the water and place one
on each side of the bagel

BREAKFAST SMOOTHIE

WHAT YOU NEED

½ avocado

Handful of baby spinach

1 small banana

Handful of blueberries

1 dessert spoon chia seeds

4 whole almonds

300ml almond milk (or any milk alternative of your choice)

THE FUN PART

Chop the avocado into chinks and place into smoothie maker

Add all the other ingredients, pouring the milk over the top

Blend until smooth and enjoy

LUNCH

GREEK SALAD

WHAT YOU NEED	THE FUN PART
200G Arla Apetina Feta cheese (or dairy free alternative)	Chop the Feta cheese into cubes
	Slice the cucumber into thin strips
15 baby tomatoes	Slice the baby tomatoes into halves
1 cucumber	
	Slice the onion into small, thin strips
1 medium red onion	
	Combine all the above ingredients into a large bowl
1 tablespoon balsamic vinegar	
2 tablespoons Extra virgin olive oil	Add the olive oil, balsamic vinegar and oregano
2 teaspoons Oregano	Stir gently to coat all the ingredients

Great served as a meal for lunch or a side dish with a main meal

CHORIZO AND RED PEPPER FRITTATA

WHAT YOU NEED

1 large white potato (peeled)

4 free range eggs (whisked)

100g Fage Total Greek yoghurt
(or dairy free alternative)

1 large red bell pepper

1 small chorizo sausage

1 teaspoon black pepper

1 teaspoon dried chives

Grated cheddar cheese
(or dairy free soya cheese alternative)

THE FUN PART

Stir the Greek yoghurt into the whisked eggs
and stir until smooth

Stir the black pepper and chives into the egg
and yoghurt mixture

Slice the potato into thin circles, the bell
peppers into thin strips and the Chorizo
into small cubes

Cover the bottom of a flan dish with a single
layer of potatoes

Place some of the Chorizo and peppers evenly
over the potatoes

Pour over some of the egg and yoghurt mixture
to cover the potatoes

Repeat the same process, layering the same
way until the ingredients are used

Sprinkle the cheddar cheese over the top

Place in the middle of a pre-heated oven, gas
mark 5 and cook for 30 minutes, or until egg is
set

BUTTERNUT SQUASH AND CHILLI SOUP

WHAT YOU NEED

1 large butternut squash

1 Kallo vegetable stock cube

1 teaspoon red chilli flakes

½ teaspoon cumin powder

½ teaspoon chilli powder

500ml almond milk
(or any milk alternative of your choice)

THE FUN PART

Cut the butternut squash in half and scoop out the seeds

Place the butternut squash on a baking sheet

Drizzle a little olive oil over the butternut squash

Sprinkle the chilli flakes, cumin powder and chilli powder evenly over the butternut squash

Cover with kitchen foil and cook in a pre-heated oven, gas mark 6 for 30 minutes

Remove the butternut squash from the oven and leave to cool for 10 minutes

Scoop the squash from the skin and place directly into a blender

Crumble the Kallo vegetable stock into the blender and add the almond milk

Blend until smooth (add more almond milk if you want a runnier soup)

If serving straight away, transfer the soup into a saucepan and simmer on a medium heat for 2 minutes

If making to use later, transfer the soup into an airtight container. Leave to cool completely before storing in a fridge. *Use within three days of making*

Serve with a crusty wholemeal or gluten free bun

TUNA SALAD
Serves 4

WHAT YOU NEED

½ bag of mixed salad leaves

½ cucumber

1 small red onion

10 baby tomatoes (halved)

4 pickled beetroots

2 sticks of celery

500g Fage Total Greek yoghurt
(or dairy free alternative)

2 x 160g tins of tuna in spring water

4 free range eggs (hard boiled)

THE FUN PART

Chop the mixed salad leaves and place in a salad bowl

Cut the cucumber in cubes

Slice the onion into thin strips

Cut the beetroot into cubes

Slice the celery sticks

Drain the tins of tuna

Add each of the above ingredients to the salad bowl with the mixed leaves and toss

Stir the Greek yoghurt through the salad mix to coat all the ingredients

Serve with the hard- boiled egg, halved
Or inside a crispy jacket potato if having as a dinner

FRENCH SPINACH TOAST WITH POACHED EGG & FETA

WHAT YOU NEED

3 free range eggs

Handful of baby spinach

2 slices of wholemeal bread
(or gluten free bread)

100g Arla Apetina Feta cheese
(or dairy free alternative)

200ml Almond milk
(or milk alternative of your choice)

Dried oregano

THE FUN PART

In a blender, mix 1 egg, spinach and
almond milk

Lay the bread onto a grill and pour the blended
mixture evenly over the bread, allowing the
mixture to absorb into the bread

Crumble the Feta cheese evenly between the
slices of bread

Sprinkle with the dried oregano (to taste)

Place the bread under a medium grill and until
the bread start to crisp (you will see the edges
browning)

Meanwhile, place the other two eggs into a
deep pan of boiling water and leave to poach
for 3 minutes. Ensure eggs are cooked before
removing from water (you can soft boil the eggs
if preferred)

Remove the toast from grill, place on a plate
and lay one egg on each of the slices

STUFFED MUSHROOM WITH ROCKET SALAD

WHAT YOU NEED

2 large chestnut mushrooms

1 slice quality ham

1 free range egg

Grated mozzarella cheese
(Tofu is a great alternative)

Dried oregano

½ bag rocket salad

Juice of ½ lemon

THE FUN PART

Remove the centre of the mushroom and place the mushrooms onto a baking tray

Slice the ham and divide equally between the the mushrooms

Whisk the egg and pour into the mushrooms

Sprinkle the egg mix with mozzarella cheese

Sprinkle the oregano over the cheese

Bake in a pre-heated oven, gas mark 6 for 20 minutes, or until egg is set

While the mushrooms are cooking, place the rocket into a bowl

Squeeze the lemon juice over the rocket and toss

Serve the mushrooms on the rocket salad

Two mushrooms per serving as a lunch, or one mushroom per serving as part of a main meal

GREEK CHICKEN PITTA POCKETS

WHAT YOU NEED | THE FUN PART

2 skinless chicken breasts

Slice the chicken breast into strips

2 wholemeal pitta breads
(or gluten free pitta breads)

heat the olive oil in a pan and add the
garlic powder and oregano

Extra virgin olive oil

Add the chicken to the pan stir to coat the
chicken strips with the oil

Juice of ½ a lemon

Add the lemon juice to the pan

2 teaspoons Oregano

Leave the chicken over a medium heat for
20-25 minutes or until chicken is cooked
thoroughly

1 teaspoon garlic powder

4 slices Halloumi
(Tofu is a great alternative)

While chicken is cooking, place the halloumi
on a griddle and cook for 2 minutes each side

Mixed lettuce leaves

Place the pitta breads in a pre-heated oven,
gas mark 5 and cook for 10 minutes, until soft
and risen

Remove the pitta breads from the oven and
with a sharp knife, slice to create a pocket,
being careful not to burn yourself

Place a handful of salad leaves into the pitta
pocket

Place the chicken into the pitta pocket,
distributing the chicken evenly

Place 2 slices of halloumi on top of the chicken

Tastes great with our Tzsasiki (in 'extras' recipes)

ONE BOWL MIXED LEAF BEETROOT SALAD WITH FETA, HAM AND EGG
Each bowl serves one

WHAT YOU NEED

½ bag of mixed leaves

2 hard-boiled eggs

2 slices of quality ham

4 pickled beetroots

100g Arla Apetina Feta cheese
(or dairy free alternative)

1 stick celery

¼ cucumber

5 baby tomatoes

1 small red onion

2 teaspoons balsamic vinegar

1 teaspoon oregano

THE FUN PART

Place the mixed leaves in a serving bowl

Slice the beetroots into quarters, add to
the mixed leaves

Cut the Feta into cubes, add to the mixed leaves

Slice the celery, add to the mixed leaves

Slice the cucumber into chunks, add to the
mixed leaves

Slice the onion into thick slices

Toss the contents of the bowl together

Drizzle the balsamic vinegar over the salad

Sprinkle the oregano over the salad

Roll the ham into tubes and place over the bowl

Slice the eggs in half and position around the
edge of the bowl

Place the tomatoes on top of the salad

Eat straight from the bowl

DINNER

CHILLI CON CARNE Y CHILLI SIN CARNE

WHAT YOU NEED

1 pound lean beef mince
or 1 pound Quorn mince

2 tins of kidney beans
(drained and rinsed under cold water)

2 tins of chopped tomatoes

1 large onion
(finely chopped)

Chilli powder (to taste)

1 carton Passata

1 tablespoon tomato puree

1 heaped tablespoon marmite

3 squares 70% dark chocolate

Olive oil

Basmati rice
(Uncle Bens ready in 2 minutes rice is
perfect for a quick mid-week solution)
Allow half a bag per person

THE FUN PART

In a large pan, heat the olive oil and brown the
beef mince (or Quorn mince)

Once browned, drain off any excess liquid,
return to the heat and add the onions

Pour in the tinned chopped tomatoes and
Kidneys beans and stir through

Add the carton of passata and stir

Add the Marmite and stir

Add the tomato puree and stir

Add the chilli powder gradually, until the
desired heat is achieved

Add the dark chocolate and stir until melted

Leave to simmer on a low heat for 20 minutes,
stirring occasionally

Add more chilli powder if desired

Remove from heat and leave to stand

Cook rice as per packet instructions

Serve with grated cheese or a blob of Fage Total Greek yoghurt
(or dairy free cheese or yoghurt alternatives)

Any chilli left can be kept in the fridge to use the next day or frozen for future meals
(do not freeze if cooked using beef mince that had previously been frozen)

CHICKEN THAI GREEN CURRY
Serves 4

WHAT YOU NEED

4 skinless chicken breasts

1 can of coconut milk

1 red bell pepper

1 green pepper

1 jar Thai green curry paste

Handful baby corns

Basmati Rice
(Uncle Bens Ready in 2 Minutes rice is perfect for a quick mid-week meal solution) Allow ½ a bag per person

Virgin coconut oil

THE FUN PART

Cut chicken breasts into strips

Cut bell peppers into strips

Cut the baby corn into half's

Combine 2 teaspoons of Thai green curry paste and 1 heaped teaspoon of coconut oil in a large pan and heat

Add the chicken strips to the pan and stir to coat with the curry paste

Cook over a medium heat for 5 minutes, stirring occasionally

Add more curry paste if desired, until preferred spice is achieved

Add the peppers and baby corn and simmer over a low heat for 20 minutes, stirring occasionally

In a separate pan, melt a teaspoon of coconut oil in a frying pan

Empty the rice into the pan and stir fry for 2 minutes or until rice is cooked

Divide the rice into your serving bowls

Remove the curry from the heat, ensuring the chicken is cooked thoroughly

Divide the curry between your serving bowls, serving directly over the rice

MEATBALLS AND SPAGHETTI

YOU WILL NEED

1 pound lean beef mince

1 egg (whisked)

2 cartons passata

2 desert spoons tomato puree

2 dessert spoons lazy garlic

1 white onion

1 desert spoon basil

1 desert spoon oregano

Black pepper

1 packet brown rice spaghetti

THE FUN PART

For the meatballs:

Place the beef mince in a large bowl

Season the minced beef with a pinch of salt and black pepper

Pour the egg into the minced beef and combine with your hands

Scoop out a palm-full of the minced beef and using the palm of your hands, roll into balls

Place the meatballs into a fridge until needed

For the Sauce:

Finely chop the onions

Pour both cartons of passata into a large pan over a low heat

Add the onion to the pan

Stir the tomato puree into the passata

Add the garlic, oregano and basil and stir

Remove meatballs from the fridge and place gently into sauce

Simmer on a medium heat for 30 minutes, or until meatballs are cooked thoroughly, stirring gently occasionally

Cook brown rice spaghetti as per packet instructions

Drain the spaghetti and place in a bowl, creating a crater in the middle

Remove the meatballs from the heat and place meatballs in the spaghetti crater (allow 5 meatballs per adult serving)

CHILLI PENNE WITH SPINACH AND FETA

WHAT YOU NEED

1 mug full of brown rice penne
(1 mug per person)

8 baby tomatoes

1 handful baby spinach

2 teaspoons chilli powder

200 grams Arla Apetina classic Feta cheese
(cut into cubes)
(or dairy free alternative)

1 dessert spoon extra virgin olive oil

THE FUN PART

Cook the brown rice Penne as per packet instructions, drain and set aside

heat the olive oil in a frying pan with the chilli powder and stir

Pour the cooked brown rice Penne into the pan and stir to coat with the chilli oil

Add the baby tomatoes and spinach and cook over a low heat until spinach is wilted

Add the Feta cheese and stir through until the Feta starts to soften and coat the Penne

Remove from heat and serve immediately

Serve with crunchy green salad

CHICKEN KORMA
Serves 4

WHAT YOU NEED

4 skinless chicken breasts
(Cut into chunks)

2 tablespoons of Korma curry powder

100g desiccated coconut

100g almond flakes

1000g Fage Total Greek yoghurt
(or dairy free alternative)

Basmati rice
(Uncle Bens Ready in 2 Minutes rice
is ideal for a quick mid-week
meal solution) Allow ½ a bag per person

THE FUN PART

Pour the Greek yoghurt into a large pan and place over a low heat

Stir the Korma curry powder into the yoghurt and continue to stir until powder is dissolved

Add the desiccated coconut to the pan

Crumble the almonds flakes into the pan and stir well

Add the chicken and stir, ensuring the chicken is well coated

Simmer on a medium heat for 30 minutes or until chicken is thoroughly cooked

Cook rice as packet instructions and share the evenly between 4 servings

Divide the chicken korma next to the rice

SIMPLE KEDGEREE
Serves 4

3 fillets of cod or mackerel fillets

Cover the fish in kitchen foil and cook in a pre-heated oven, gas mark 6, for 10 minutes

Basmati rice
(Uncle Bens Ready in 2 Minutes rice is ideal for a quick mid-week meal solution)
Allow 2 bags for this recipe

Heat the olive oil in a large pan

1 mugful frozen peas

Pour the rice into the pan and stir to separate the grains

1 white onion (finely chopped)

Add the cooked fish to the rice and stir through to crumble the fish

1 dessert spoon oregano

Add the peas and onions and stir again

1 dessert spoon cumin

Add the oregano and cumin

Juice of 1 lemon

Cook over a low heat for 10 minutes, stirring occasionally

4 free range eggs (hard boiled)

Remove from heat and squeeze lemon juice over the top

Extra virgin olive oil

Divide between 4 servings, arranging an egg (quartered) onto each serving

Serve with a mixed leaf salad

BEEF STROGANOFF
Serves 4

WHAT YOU NEED

2 large rump steaks

1 green bell pepper

1 red bell pepper

1 white onion

1 dessert spoon paprika

2 teaspoons ground black pepper

2 tablespoons lazy garlic

1kg Total Greek yoghurt
(or dairy free alternative)

Basmati rice
(Uncle bens Ready in 2 Minutes rice is
ideal for a quick mid-week meal solution)
Allow ½ bag per person

THE FUN PART

Cut the steaks into strips and set aside

Slice the bells peppers into strips

Slice the onion into thin strips

In a large pan, heat the Greek yoghurt over
a medium heat

Add the lazy garlic to the pan and stir through

Add the paprika and black pepper and stir until
the paprika has dissolved

Place the steak into the pan and stir, ensuring all
steak is covered by the sauce

Add peppers and onion and stir

Leave to simmer on a medium heat for
20 minutes, stirring occasionally

Cook the rice as per the packet instructions and
divide between 4 servings

Ensure the steak is cooked thoroughly and
divide the stroganoff between the 4 servings

CHARGRILLED CHICKEN WITH BROCCOLI AND HALOUMI STACK
Serves 4

WHAT YOU NEED

4 skinless chicken breasts

1 pack of Haloumi (sliced)
(Tofu is a great alternative)

12 stems of baby stem broccoli

20 baby potatoes

THE FUN PART

Before starting, place the baby potatoes into a pre-heated oven, gas mark 6, and cook for 25-30 minutes

Individually cover the chicken breasts in cling film and using a rolling pin, hit until flattened to approximately ½ inch thick

Heat a dry griddle pan over a medium heat

Place each of the chicken breasts into the griddle and cook for 5 minutes on each side (ensure chicken is cooked thoroughly before removing from heat)

Place chicken to rest on serving plates

Replace the griddle pan to the heat

Place 8 slices of the Haloumi to the griddle and cook for 2 minutes on each

While the Haloumi is cooking, place the broccoli in a microwave container and steam in microwave for 60 seconds

Remove the broccoli from the microwave and place 2 stems onto each of the chicken escalope's

Remove the Haloumi from heat and stack 2 slices on top of the chicken and broccoli

Remove the baby potatoes from the oven and serve 5 potatoes per serving

Serve with Greek Salad

CHICKEN CORDON BLEU
Serves 4

4 skinless chicken breasts

4 slices quality ham

4 white mushrooms (thinly sliced)

Grated mozzarella or Gouda cheese
(or dairy free cheese alternative)

12 cocktail sticks

Slice each of the chicken breasts end to end to
to create a pocket

Place 1 slice of ham inside each of the chicken
breast pockets

Divide the mushrooms between the chicken
breasts, placing them inside the pockets

Push a palm-full of cheese into each of the
chicken pockets

Using 4 cocktail sticks per chicken breast, thread
the cocktail sticks along the length of each of
the chicken breasts to hold the pockets together

Place the chicken breasts on to a flat tray lined
with greaseproof paper

Place in a pre-heated oven, gas mark 5 for 30
minutes or until chicken is cooked throughout
before removing from oven

Serve with homemade oven chips and crunchy green salad and peas

CHICKEN NUGGETS

WHAT YOU NEED

4 skinless chicken breasts
(you can use Quorn 'chicken')

2 free range eggs (whisked)

Wholemeal flour
(or gluten free flour)

1 tea spoon ground black pepper

1 teaspoon paprika

1 teaspoon garlic powder

4 wholemeal bread rolls
(or gluten free rolls)

Olive Oil

THE FUN PART

Before you start, place the wholemeal bread rolls into a blender and mill into breadcrumbs

Cut the chicken into chunks

Place the whisked eggs into a bowl

Place the wholemeal flour into a bowl

Mix the black pepper, paprika and garlic powder into the wholemeal breadcrumbs and place Into a bowl

Dip each of the chicken chunks first into the flour, then into the egg then coat well with the breadcrumbs

Heat some olive oil on a large flat oven tray in a pre-heated oven, gas mark 5. Remove the tray from the oven and place the coated chicken nuggets directly onto the flat tray

Cook in the middle of the pre-heated oven, gas mark 5 for 25 minutes, turning once. Ensure chicken is cooked thoroughly before removing From oven

Serve with homemade oven chips, crunchy salad and sweetcorn

FISH FINGERS

WHAT YOU NEED

4 Cod Fillets

2 free range eggs (whisked)

Wholemeal flour
(or gluten free flour)

1 tea spoon ground black pepper

4 wholemeal bread rolls
(or gluten free rolls)

THE FUN PART

Cut fish into fingers approximately 1 inch thick

Follow the same steps as chicken nuggets recipe (above) excluding the garlic powder and paprika

Serve with sweet potato wedges and peas

CHILLI BEEF STUFFED BELL PEPPERS
Serves 4

WHAT YOU NEED

1 pound lean beef mince beef
(you can use Quorn mince)

4 large red bell peppers

2 teaspoons chilli powder

2 teaspoons garlic powder

1 teaspoon ground black pepper

1 white onion (finely chopped)

1 mugful of peas

250grams brown basmati rice
(Uncle Bens Ready in 2 Minutes is
perfect for a quick mid-week meal solution)

Grated cheddar cheese
(or dairy free cheese alternative)

Extra virgin olive oil

THE FUN PART

Cut the top off each of the bell peppers and
remove the seeds. Set peppers aside

Heat the olive oil in a large pan and brown the
mince beef

Add the onion and peas and stir

Stir through the rice

Add the chilli powder, garlic powder and black
pepper

Remove the beef mixture from the heat

Place each of the bell pepper onto a flat tray,
lined with grease-proof paper, ensuring they
stand upright

Using a spoon, stuff each of the bell peppers
with the beef mix, filling each one to the top.
Pack down to fill the peppers tight

Sprinkle a little of the grated cheddar on top of
each of the stuffed bell peppers

Place the stuffed peppers in the centre of a pre-
heated oven, gas mark 5 and cook for 30
minutes

Serve with a Greek salad

FAKE-A-WAY PIZZA

WHAT YOU NEED

1 pound wholemeal self-raising flour
(or gluten free self-raising flour)

2 teaspoons baking powder

4oz butter (room temperature)
(or dairy free butter alternative)

Almond milk
(or milk alternative of your choice)

1 dessert spoon of Passata

Grated mozzarella and cheddar cheese
(or dairy free cheese alternative)

2 white mushrooms

2 slices of quality ham
(alternatively, you can use toppings
of your choice)

mixed herbs

THE FUN PART

In a large bowl sift the flour and baking powder

Rub in the butter with your fingers until
breadcrumbs are formed

Pour the milk into the bowl slowly, using your
fingers to bind until a soft dough is formed
*Be careful not to pour too much milk, the dough
does not want to be wet*

Knead the dough for a couple of minutes

Sprinkle a little flour onto the worktops and
Roll the pizza dough out into an oblong

Transfer the pizza dough onto a pizza tray

Spread the passata evenly over the pizza dough

Place the ham and mushrooms (or toppings of
of your choice) evenly over the pizza dough

Sprinkle the grated mozzarella and cheddar
cheese generously over the top

Sprinkle with mixed herbs

Place in the centre of a pre-heated over, gas
mark 5 for 20 – 25 minutes, ensuring the pizza is
piping hot and cooked throughout before
removing from oven

BAKED COD WITH MEDITEREAN VEGETABLES AND BAKED EGG
Serves 4

4 cod fillets

4 handfuls broccoli florets

4 handfuls baby carrots

8 beetroots (quartered)

10 baby tomatoes

2 courgettes (thickly sliced)

4 free range eggs

Extra virgin olive oil

1 dessert spoon balsamic vinegar

1 dessert spoon oregano

Juice of ½ a lemon

4 free range eggs

Place all the vegetables into an oven-proof dish

Drizzle with a little olive oil

Add The balsamic vinegar and oregano and mix to coat the vegetables

Cover and cook in a pre-heated oven, gas mark 6, for 25 minutes

Place the cod fillets onto kitchen foil

Sprinkle lightly with oregano

Drizzle the lemon juice evenly over each of cod fillets

Fold the kitchen foil to create a pocket

Place in a pre-heated oven, gas mark 6, for 20 minutes

Remove the tray of vegetables from the oven

Create 4 craters in the tray of vegetables, by pushing some of the vegetables to the side

Crack one egg into each of the craters

Return the tray to the oven, uncovered for a further 10 minutes, or until egg whites have set

Serve the vegetables evenly between 4 servings, ensuring there is one egg per serving

Lay one cod fillet onto each of the servings

DESSERT

GREEK VOLCANO
Serves 2

WHAT YOU NEED

500g Fage Total Greek Yoghurt
(or dairy free alternative)

2 handfuls blueberries

2 handfuls halved strawberries

1 handful chopped hazelnuts

Squeezy honey

THE FUN PART

Cover the bottom of two dessert bowls with a layer of the Greek yoghurt

Place one handful of the blueberries into each of the bowls, covering the yoghurt layer

Spoon in another layer of the Greek yoghurt into each of the bowls, covering the blueberries

Place a handful of the quartered strawberries into each of the bowls, covering the yoghurt layer

Spoon in another layer of the Greek yoghurt into each of the bowls, covering the strawberries

Divide the handful of chopped hazelnuts between the two bowls, sprinkling evenly over the Greek yoghurt

Squeeze a little honey over the hazelnuts

CHOCOLATE AND WALNUT BROWNIE

WHAT YOU NEED

100g chopped walnuts

20 pitted dates
chopped into small pieces

1 dessert spoon cocoa powder
(raw cacao powder also works but
will give a more intense cocoa flavour)

½ teaspoon good quality instant coffee
powder

1 pinch of sea salt

THE FUN PART

Place half the walnuts into a blender and mill
until finely ground

Add the coca powder, coffee and sea salt
to the blender and pulse to combine

Add small handfuls of the dates a time, to the
blender and blend until a dough is formed. You
may need to add more dates or small amounts
of water to achieve a dough that holds together
when held in your hands

Place the brownie dough into a shallow cake
tin, lined with grease-proof paper and press
down evenly firmly

Scatter the remaining walnuts on top of the
brownie dough and press down firmly until they
are set in place

Place in the fridge and chill until firm (at least 2
hours) before turning out onto a flat surface

Cut the brownies into squares or fingers and
enjoy

Store brownies in an airtight container to keep fresh
They will keep in the fridge for 2 weeks or a freezer for 2 months

MILLIONAIRES SHORTBREAD
Serves 12

WHAT YOU NEED

130g porridge oats
(gluten free if desired)

45g coconut oil
plus, additional 1 teaspoon coconut oil

50g honey

1 banana

70g smooth Whole Earth peanut butter

180g partly dried figs

50g dark chocolate (at least 70% cocoa)

THE FUN PART

For the base:
Place the porridge oats into a blender and
mill into a flour

Melt 36g of coconut oil in a microwave for
30 seconds and add to the blender with the
oats

Add the honey to the blender and blend to
combine

Transfer to a cake tin, lined with grease-proof
paper and pack mixture down evenly

Place in a freezer

For the Middle layer:
Place the banana into a blender

Chop the figs into quarters and add to the
blender with the peanut butter

Melt 10g of the coconut oil in a microwave for
30 seconds and add to the blender and blend
until smooth

Take the bottom layer out of the freezer and
spoon the middle layer evenly over the top then
return to the freezer

For the top layer:
Melt the dark chocolate in a microwave until
melted, stirring every 15 seconds

Stir in the teaspoon of coconut oil

Remove the tin from the freezer and pour the
melted chocolate over the top

Return to the freezer for two

Carefully lift onto a flat surface and slice into 12
squares

60 SECOND VANILLA CAKE
1 ramakin per serving

WHAT YOU NEED

THE FUN PART

1 free range egg

Crack the egg into a ramakin (or mug) and whisk

3 tablespoons ground almonds

Stir the ground almonds into the egg until completely mixed

1 tablespoon maple syrup

1 teaspoon vanilla essence

Add the maple syrup and vanilla essence and mix well

1 tablespoon dark chocolate chips

Add the dark chocolate chips and mix well

Place in a microwave and cook for 1 minute or until a fork comes out clean

serve with vanilla nice cream

VANILLA NICE CREAM
Serves 4

WHAT YOU NEED

THE FUN PART

4 frozen bananas

Chop the bananas into chunks

2 tablespoons maple syrup

Place all the ingredients together into a blender

½ teaspoon cinnamon

Blend until a smooth, creamy texture is formed

1 teaspoon vanilla essence or vanilla paste

Serve immediately

KIWI ICE-CREAM

WHAT YOU NEED

6 Kiwi fruits

250g Fage Total Greek yoghurt
(or dairy free alternative)

Juice of 1 lime

THE FUN PART

Chop the kiwi fruits into chunks, place
into an airtight container and freeze

Place the Greek yoghurt into a blender
and add the frozen kiwi fruit chunks

Squeeze the lemon juice into the blender and
blend until a smooth consistency is formed

Spoon mixture back into the airtight container
and place in freezer until frozen

Remove once again from the freezer and tip out
onto a flat surface

Cut into cubes

Place the cubes into a blender and blend until a
creamy texture is re-formed

Spoon back into the airtight container and
freeze until ready to serve

CHOCOLATE MUFFINS
For 6 muffins

WHAT YOU NEED

4 large purple sweet potatoes
mashed and left to go cold
(if you can't get purple sweet potatoes,
sweet potatoes will be fine to use)

1 large free range egg (whisked)

1 tablespoon raw cacao powder

1 handful dried mixed fruit

1 dessert spoon coconut sugar

2 dessert spoon vanilla essence
or vanilla paste

200g unsalted cashew nuts
(softened in water for
2 hours before using)

Desiccated coconut (for decoration)

2 teaspoons cinnamon

1 large date (pitted)

1 teaspoon maple syrup

Juice of 1 lemon

THE FUN PART

For the muffins:
Place the mashed sweet potato into a large mixing bowl

Pour in the egg and mix and combine

Add the cacao powder, mixed dried fruit, coconut sugar and dessert spoon of vanilla essence and mix well

Spoon the mixture evenly between the muffin cases, filling each once to the top

Place in the middle of a pre-heated oven, gas mark 5 for 35 minutes, or until a fork comes out clean

Remove from oven and leave to cool completely

For the frosting:
Drain the cashews and place in a blender

Add the cinnamon, date, 1 dessert spoon of vanilla essence, maple syrup and lemon juice

Blend until a stiff, creamy consistency is formed
You may need to add a little water to the blender if the mixture thickens too much

Spoon or pipe the cashew frosting onto the muffins, creating a high frosting each muffin

Sprinkle each muffin with a little desiccated coconut

STRAWBERRY CHEESECAKE BALLS
Makes 10

WHAT YOU NEED

250g cream cheese
(or dairy free cream cheese alternative)

1 teaspoon vanilla bean paste

1 ½ tablespoons maple syrup

10 small strawberries

50g ground almonds

THE FUN PART

Place the cream cheese into a mixing bowl

Add the vanilla bean and maple syrup and mix well

Spoon the mixture into an ice cube tray, filling mould half way high (you can use a cake-pop mould if preferred)

Place one strawberry into each of the moulds, pushing gently into the cream cheese mix

Take the remaining cream cheese mixture and place over each of the strawberries, ensuring to cover the strawberries completely

Place in the freezer for two hours

Meanwhile, gently heat a dry pan on a low heat and add the ground almonds to toast evenly

Set the toasted ground almonds aside to cool

Remove the cheesecakes from the freezer and one at a time, gently roll in the palm of your hands to create balls

Roll each of the cheesecake balls into the toasted ground almonds, then roll in the palm of your hands once again before rolling once more in the toasted ground almonds

Repeat this process with each of the cheesecake balls

Store in the fridge until ready to serve

CHILDREN'S SNACKS AND SIDES

WHOLEMEAL LOAF

WHAT YOU NEED

500g strong wholemeal bread flour

1 teaspoon sea salt

1 sachet easy-bake yeast

300ml warm water

2 tablespoons extra virgin olive oil

THE FUN PART

In a large mixing bowl, mix the wholemeal bread flour with the sea salt and easy-bake yeast

In a separate bowl, mix the water with the extra virgin olive oil

Pour the water and oil mixture into the bowl with the flour and mix until a dough is formed

Knead the dough WITH OILED HANDS for 10 minutes

Shape the dough into a loaf or into buns and place onto a flat, oiled tray

Cover the dough and store in a warm place for one hour, or until the dough has doubled in size (an airing cupboard is ideal for this)

Cook in the middle of a pre-heated over, gas mark 6 for 30 minutes – you can check to make sure bread is cooked by tapping it with your knuckles. If the bread sounds hollow, it is cooked

GLUTEN AND WHEAT FREE LOAF

WHAT YOU NEED

500g gluten and wheat free bread flour

1 teaspoon sea salt

1 sachet easy-bake yeast

300ml warm water

2 tablespoons extra virgin olive oil

THE FUN PART

Follow the same method as the wholemeal loaf, above, replacing the wholemeal bread flour with the gluten and wheat free bread flour

STRAWBERRY AND COCONUT JAM

WHAT YOU NEED

1 punnet of strawberries

3 dessert spoons desiccated coconut

Juice of one lemon

THE FUN PART

Chop the strawberries into quarters and heat
In a saucepan over a medium heat, stirring
constantly

Once the strawberries have mushed and starts
to turn to a liquid, add the desiccated coconut
and lemon juice and continue stirring until a
smooth, thick consistency is achieved

Pour the jam into a jar and set aside to cool

Once cooled, cover and store in the fridge

This will store in a fridge for 4 days

TZATZIKI

WHAT YOU NEED

500g Fage Total Greek yoghurt
(or dairy free alternative)

3 heaped teaspoons lazy garlic

1 cucumber

1 dessert spoon mint sauce

THE FUN PART

Tip the Greek yoghurt into a bowl

Stir in the lazy garlic and mint sauce

Grate the outer layer of the cucumber,
(discard the watery middle section) and
stir through the Greek yoghurt mix

Store in a fridge until ready to use

Use within 3 days

GRANOLA BARS
Makes 12 squares

WHAT YOU NEED
225g porridge oats
(gluten free if preferred)

100g mixed seeds

1 dessert spoon sultanas

4 dried apricots (cut into chunks)

1 dessert spoon coconut sugar

1 dessert spoon maple syrup

1 dessert spoon vanilla essence or paste

1 large free range egg (whisked)

2 dessert spoons virgin coconut oil
(melted)

THE FUN PART
Place the porridge oats into a large mixing bowl

Add the mixed seeds, sultanas, dried apricots and coconut sugar and mix well

Add the egg to the bowl and mix well

Pour in the maple syrup, vanilla essence and melted coconut oil and stir well

Pour the mixture out into a high-sided baking tray, lined with grease-proof paper

Pack down until the mixture is packed tight, evenly across the tray

Bake in a pre-heated oven, gas mark 6 for 25 minutes

Remove from oven and leave to cool down

Turn out onto a flat surface and slice into squares

BEETROOT SALAD

WHAT YOU NEED
8 pickled beetroots

1 small white onion

2 teaspoons of garlic powder

1 dessert spoon of balsamic vinegar

THE FUN PART
Slice the beetroot into small chunks and place in a bowl

Slice the onion into small, thin slices and and add to the beetroot

Add the garlic powder and balsamic vinegar and stir well

Place in fridge until ready to serve

LENTIL PATE

WHAT YOU NEED

1 mug of red lentils

1 dessert spoon medium curry powder

1 teaspoon lazy garlic

1 Kallo vegetable stock cube

1 onion (chopped)

1 teaspoon mango chutney

1 free range egg (whisked)

1 dessert spoon almond milk
(or milk alternative of your choice)

THE FUN PART

Place the lentils into a pan of water over a medium heat

Add the onion, garlic and curry powder and simmer for 15-20 minutes

Drain and set aside to cool

Once cool, place the lentil mix into a blender

Add the egg and mango chutney and blend, adding a little of the milk to combine

Transfer the lentil mix into a loaf tin, greased with olive oil

Cover with kitchen foil and cook in a pre-heated oven, gas mark 5 for 35-40 minutes or until firm to touch

OVEN CHIPS (the whole family can enjoy)
4 portions

WHAT YOU NEED

4 medium white potatoes

Extra virgin olive oil

Pinch of sea salt

THE FUN PART

Cut each of the potatoes in half, then slice each half into chip strips

Drizzle a little oil onto a flat oven tray and heat in a pre-heated oven, gas mark 5, for 5 minutes

Lay a single layer of the potatoes onto the heated tray

Drizzle the potatoes with a little olive oil and sprinkle with a little sea salt

Return tray to the oven and cook for 35 minutes or until chips are golden brown

10

TIME TO START

believe in yourself

Now all that is left to do is take some photos and take your measurements. Nothing will motivate you more than a visual reminder of your own progress. Looking back at your 'before' photos and watching your measurements shrink will be the best source of personal motivation for you.

Ask someone to take these photos for you, or alternatively, stand in front of a full-length mirror and take three photos; one front view, one standing sideways and one rear view. Remember to date these photos.

Now grab your tape measure and take your measurements, filling in the chart within this book. The start date will be the date that you are literally ready to start following L.I.F.E. Fit - The Process entirely. So, your kitchen has been stripped of the ready-made and processed foods, the sugary foods that will tempt you are removed, and you have been shopping and are fully stocked up with the foods you need to follow the menus above.

The second date will be 12 weeks from your start date and the third date will be 24 weeks from your start date. It is important to remember that the 24-week marker does not signify the end of L.I.F.E. Fit. It is simply a marker of your 24-weeks progress. L.I.F.E. Fit - The Process is designed to give you principles to follow for a healthy lifestyle and to that effect, there is no 'end' date.

START DATE: _____

Weight: _____

Neck: _____ Chest:_____

Waist: _____ Hips:_____

R.Arm: _____ Thigh:_____

12 WEEKS: _____

Weight: _____

Neck: _____ Chest:_____

Waist: _____ Hips:_____

R.Arm: _____ Thigh:_____

DIFFERENCE: Neck: _____ Chest: _____

Waist: _____ Hips: _____ R.Arm:_____Thigh: _____

RESULTS: Total Inches Lost:_____ Total Weight Lost: _____

24 WEEKS: _____

Weight: _____

Neck: _____ Chest:_____

Waist: _____ Hips: _____

R.Arm: _____ Thigh:_____

DIFFERENCE: Neck: _____ Chest: _____

Waist: _____ Hips: _____ R.Arm:_____ Right Thigh: _____

RESULTS: Total Inches Lost: _____   Total Weight Lost: _____

111

Okay, this is where I stop talking and you start doing. Before you go, there is one thing you must do, continuously…. BELIEVE!

Now, with that said, go and be fabulous.

EXERCISE

HOME GYM WORKOUT: CORE   (Monday)

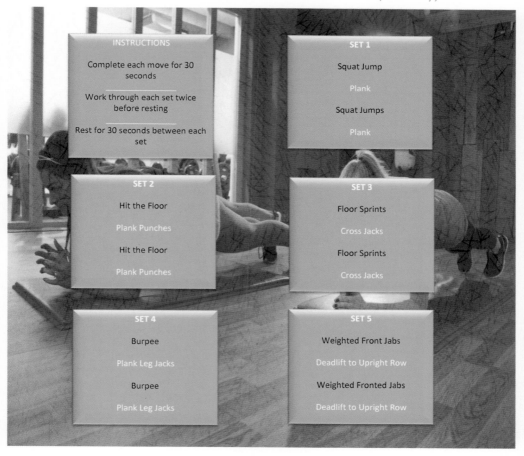

INSTRUCTIONS

Complete each move for 30 seconds

Work through each set twice before resting

Rest for 30 seconds between each set

SET 1

Squat Jump

Plank

Squat Jumps

Plank

SET 2

Hit the Floor

Plank Punches

Hit the Floor

Plank Punches

SET 3

Floor Sprints

Cross Jacks

Floor Sprints

Cross Jacks

SET 4

Burpee

Plank Leg Jacks

Burpee

Plank Leg Jacks

SET 5

Weighted Front Jabs

Deadlift to Upright Row

Weighted Fronted Jabs

Deadlift to Upright Row

EXERCISES

HOME GYM WORKOUT: **UPPER BODY** (Tuesday)

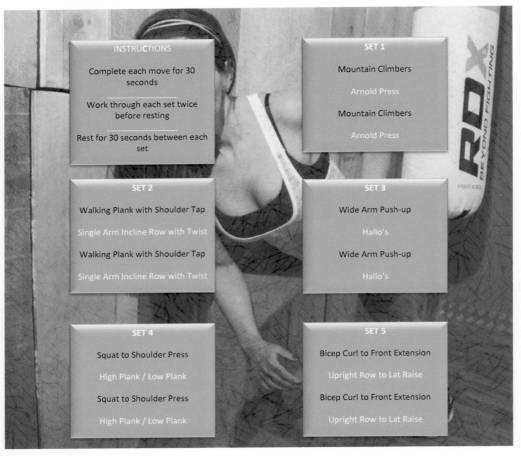

INSTRUCTIONS

Complete each move for 30 seconds

Work through each set twice before resting

Rest for 30 seconds between each set

SET 1

Mountain Climbers

Arnold Press

Mountain Climbers

Arnold Press

SET 2

Walking Plank with Shoulder Tap

Single Arm Incline Row with Twist

Walking Plank with Shoulder Tap

Single Arm Incline Row with Twist

SET 3

Wide Arm Push-up

Hallo's

Wide Arm Push-up

Hallo's

SET 4

Squat to Shoulder Press

High Plank / Low Plank

Squat to Shoulder Press

High Plank / Low Plank

SET 5

Bicep Curl to Front Extension

Upright Row to Lat Raise

Bicep Curl to Front Extension

Upright Row to Lat Raise

EXERCISES

HOME GYM WORKOUT: **ABS**   (Wednesday)

INSTRUCTIONS
Complete each move for 30 seconds
Work through each set twice before resting
Rest for 30 seconds between each set

SET 1
Jumping Jacks
Toe Taps
Jumping Jacks
Tow Taps

SET 2
Overhead High Knees
Scissors
Overhead High Knees
Scissors

SET 3
Floor Sprints
Standing Oblique Crunch
Floor Sprints
Standing Oblique Crunch

SET 4
High Knee Ankle Taps
Hand to Toe Taps
High Knee Ankle Taps
Hand to Toe Taps

SET 5
Russian Twists
Rainbow Lifts
Russian Twists
Rainbow Lifts

EXERCISES

HOME GYM WORKOUT: **LEGS & GLUTES**   (Thursday)

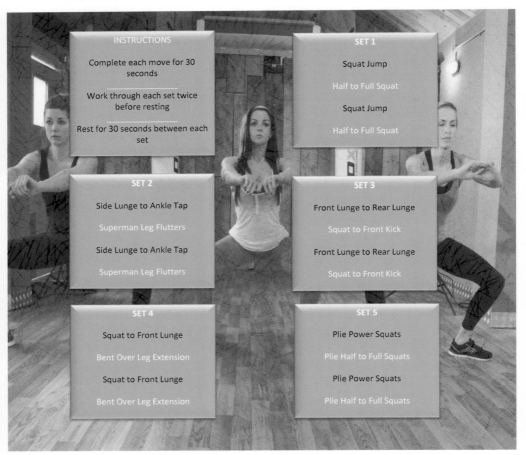

INSTRUCTIONS

Complete each move for 30 seconds

Work through each set twice before resting

Rest for 30 seconds between each set

SET 1

Squat Jump

Half to Full Squat

Squat Jump

Half to Full Squat

SET 2

Side Lunge to Ankle Tap

Superman Leg Flutters

Side Lunge to Ankle Tap

Superman Leg Flutters

SET 3

Front Lunge to Rear Lunge

Squat to Front Kick

Front Lunge to Rear Lunge

Squat to Front Kick

SET 4

Squat to Front Lunge

Bent Over Leg Extension

Squat to Front Lunge

Bent Over Leg Extension

SET 5

Plie Power Squats

Plie Half to Full Squats

Plie Power Squats

Plie Half to Full Squats

EXERCISES

HOME GYM WORKOUT: **FULL BODY** (Friday)

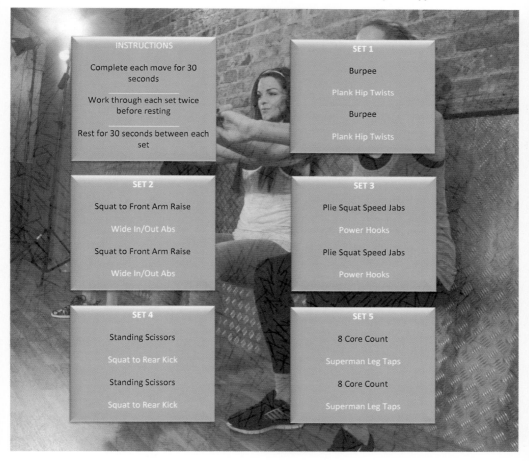

INSTRUCTIONS

Complete each move for 30 seconds

Work through each set twice before resting

Rest for 30 seconds between each set

SET 1

Burpee

Plank Hip Twists

Burpee

Plank Hip Twists

SET 2

Squat to Front Arm Raise

Wide In/Out Abs

Squat to Front Arm Raise

Wide In/Out Abs

SET 3

Plie Squat Speed Jabs

Power Hooks

Plie Squat Speed Jabs

Power Hooks

SET 4

Standing Scissors

Squat to Rear Kick

Standing Scissors

Squat to Rear Kick

SET 5

8 Core Count

Superman Leg Taps

8 Core Count

Superman Leg Taps

EXCERCISES EXPLAINED

SQUAT JUMPS

1. Stand with your feet shoulder width apart
2. Lower your body into a squat position
3. Using your arms to help propel you, jump as high as you can, with straight legs
4. As you land, bend your legs straight away so that you are landing in the staring squat position

MODIFIED
Remove the jump from the move, coming straight out of the squat into a standing position

ADVANCED
Move faster, trying to improve your personal best each time
Add ankle and/or wrist weights

PLANK

1. Lay on the floor on your front
2. Bend your arms, placing your forearms on the floor so that your elbows are directly under your shoulders
3. Support your weight onto your forearms
4. With straight legs, hold you your legs up on your toes (as you would in a push-up position)
5. Your body should remain in a straight line from shoulders to ankles
6. Hold the position by sucking your tummy in

MODIFIED
Bring your knees to rest on the floor (your knees should not be directly under your hips)

ADVANCED
Add weight to your back

HIT THE FLOOR

1. Standing with your hands down by your side

2. Step your right leg out to the side while at the same time, taking your right hand down to touch your left foot

3. Return to standing position, bringing your right leg back to starting position, while you take both hands up over your head

4. Step your left leg out to the side while at the same time, taking your left hand down to touch your right foot

5. Return to standing position, bringing your left leg back to starting position, while you take both hands up over your head

6. Repeat alternating sides at speed

MODIFIED
Move slower
Touch your shin instead of your foot

ADVANCED
Move faster
Add ankle and/or wrist weights

PLANK PUNCHES

1. Start by holding yourself in a push-up position

2. Make sure your wrists are placed directly under your shoulders

3. Lift your left arm and punch out in front of you, level with your shoulder

4. Return your left hand to the floor

5. Lift your right arm and punch out in front of you, level with your shoulder

MODIFIED
Bring your knees to rest on the floor (your knees should not be directly under your hips)

ADVANCED
Concentrate on keeping your core as still as possible
Add wrist weights

FLOOR SPRINTS

1. Starting in a push-up position, with your wrists placed directly under your shoulders

2. Hold your tummy in tight

3. Bring one knee in towards your chest, keeping your toes off the floor

4. Return this foot to starting position, while at the same time, bringing your other leg in towards your chest

5. Continue this movement in a motion mimicking running on the spot

MODIFIED
You can step the move, taking your knee in towards your chest, then return to starting position and securing your food on the floor before bringing your other knee in towards your chest

ADVANCED
Go as fast as you can
Add ankle weights
Add a resistance band around your ankles

CROSS JACKS

1. Stand with your feet shoulder width apart

2. Raise bent arms out to your side with your elbows level with your shoulders

3. Alternating knee to opposite elbow to meet in the middle, hopping as you bring your knee in and jumping back into the start position

MODIFIED
Remove the hop and jump, raising your knee to opposite elbow and stepping back into place

ADVANCED
Mover faster
Add ankle and/or wrist weights

BURPEE

1. Standing with your feet shoulder-width apart

2. Lower your body into a squat position, placing your hands on the floor in front of you

3. Holding your tummy in tight, jump both feet out, taking you into a push-up position

4. Holding your tummy in tight, jump both feet back in and taking your hands off the floor so you are back into the squat position

5. Push up through your legs, jumping in the air with your hands up over your head

6. As you land, bend your legs taking you straight back in the squat position ready to repeat the move

MODIFIED
From the squat position, step your feet out one at a time into the push-up position
Step your feet back in to the squat position
Stand up

ADVANCED
See how many burpees you can do in the allocated time, trying to beat your personal best each time
There are so many variations to the Burpee, there are no limits to what you can do with this move as your strength grows. Have fun with it

PLANK LEG JACKS

1. Starting in the plank position

2. Hold your tummy in tight

3. Jump your legs, at the same time out to the side

4. Immediately jump your legs back to the starting position

MODIFIELD
Step your legs out to the side one at a time and return them to the starting position one at a time

ADVANCED
Add ankle weights
Add a resistance band around your ankles

WEIGHTED FRONT JABS

1. Holding a light hand weight

2. Stand with your feet slightly wider than shoulder width apart, toes pointing outwards

3. Lower yourself into a plie squat

4. Hold your tummy in tight and keep your shoulders and chest up

5. Punch forward, alternating your arms, allowing your body to twist at your waist

MODIFIED
Don't use a hand weight
Move slower

ADVANCED
Use a heavier hand weight
Move faster
Sit yourself in a lower plie squat

DEADLIFT TO UPRIGHT ROW

1. Hold your hand weight in front of your body

2. Holding your tummy tight and moving from your hips, push your bottom out as you bend down, with a slight bend in your knees, lowering the weights to your ankles

3. Moving from your hips, lift the weights back to the starting position, squeezing your glutes as you lift

4. From starting position, lift the weights to your chin, raising your elbows higher than your shoulders

5. Lower the weights to starting position

6. Repeat from beginning

MODIFIED
Use lighter weights
Bend your knees more and don't lower the weights as low

ADVANCED
Use a heavier weight

MOUNTAIN CLIMBERS

1. Run on the spot, bring your knees up level with your hips (high knee)
2. At the same time, alternate your arms up above your head with a bent arm (as if you are climbing a ladder, fast)

MODIFIED
Step on the spot instead of running

ADVANCED
Perform the move as fast as you can
Add ankle and/or wrist weights

ARNOLD PRESS

1. Holding a hand weight in each hand, stand with feet shoulder width apart
2. Hold your tummy in tight
3. Hold the weights up at shoulder height
4. Push the weights above your head
5. Bring the weights back to shoulder level
6. Bring your elbows together, keeping the weights at the same height
7. Return your elbows to the starting position
8. Repeat from the beginning

MODIFIED
Use a lighter weight

ADVANCED
Use a heavier weight

WALKING PLANK WITH SHOULDER TAP

1. Start in the push-up position
2. Step your left arm and left leg to the left at the same time, for two steps
3. Lift your right hand and tap your left shoulder
4. Return your right hand to the floor
5. Step your right arm and right leg to the right at the same time, for two steps
6. Lift your left hand and tap your right shoulder
7. Repeat from beginning. Make sure you keep your body in a straight line from shoulder to ankles throughout the move

MODIFIED
Hold yourself in push-up position, keep your legs where they are and tap your left hand once to the left, then tap your right hand to the right once

ADVANCED
Add wrist and/or wrist weights

SINGLE ARM INCLINE ROW WITH TWIST

1. Hold a hand weight in your right hand
2. Bend forward, with your left leg in front and your right leg behind you
3. Support your weight with your forearm resting on your bent left leg
4. Raise your right elbow, lifting the weight to your side
5. Lower the weight by straightening your arm
6. Holding your tummy tight, with a straight arm, swing your right arm, twisting your body to the right until your hand is pointing towards the ceiling
7. With a straight arm, return to the starting position
8. Continue for the stated time before repeating on the other side

MODIFIED
Use a lighter hand weight

ADVANCED
Use a heavier hand weight

WIDE ARM PUSH-UP

1. Start in the push-up position
2. Take your hands wider than your shoulders
3. Lower yourself slowly, taking your chest to the floor, squeezing your shoulder blades together
4. Return slowly to the starting position

MODIFIED
Lower your knees to the floor (your knees should not be directly under your hips)

ADVANCED
Move slowly throughout the upward and downward motion
Add weight to your back

HALLO'S

1. Stand with your feet about one inch apart
2. Hold a hand weight in both hands under your chin with your elbows out to the side
3. Hold your tummy in tight
4. Rotate the hand weight clockwise around your head, taking it behind your head and under your chin
5. Continue clockwise for stated time before changing to anti-clockwise for stated time

MODIFIED
Use a lighter weight
Reduce your range of motion

ADVANCED
Use a heavier hand weight

SQUAT TO SHOULDER PRESS

1. Hold your hand weights, one in each hand
2. Stand with feet shoulder width apart with weights held in front of you
3. Lower yourself to a squat
4. Return to a standing position, raising the hand weights to shoulder level
5. Press the weights up over your head
6. Return the weights to shoulder level before lowering them to hold in front of you

MODIFIED
Use lighter weights

ADVANCED
Use heavier weights

HIGH PLANK / LOW PLANK

1. Start in the plank position, holding your tummy in tight
2. Starting with your left arm, raise up onto your hand
3. Raise up onto your right hand
4. Lower your left arm back down to your forearm
5. Lower your right arm back down to your forearm
6. Repeat, this time starting with your right arm

MODIDFIED
Lower your knees to the floor (your knees should not be directly under your hips)

ADVANVECD
Add weight to your back
Place a step in front of you (or face your stairs) and when you come up onto your hand, then step the same hand up onto the step before returning it to the floor then lowering onto your forearm

BICEP CURL TO FRONT EXTENSION

1. Holding a hand weight in each hand with the back of your hand facing your body, stand with feet shoulder width apart

2. Hold your tummy in tight, elbows tucked into the side of your body

3. Bend both arms, raising the hand weight up towards your shoulder

4. Lower the hand weight to starting position

5. Twist the back of your hand away from you to face the wall opposite

6. Raise both arms straight up in front of you to shoulder height

7. Return to start position, twisting the back of your hand to face your body

8. Repeat from the beginning

MODIFIED
Use a lighter weight
When lifting straight arms in front of you, don't lift as high

ADVANCED
Use a heavier weight

UPRIGHT ROW TO LAT RAISE

1. Holding a hand weight in each hand, stand with feet shoulder width apart with the back of your hand facing the wall opposite

2. Raise the weights to your chin, lifting your elbows higher than your shoulders

3. Return to the start position, twisting the back of your hands to face the walls either side of you

4. Raise your arms up to the side of you, with a bent arm, raising your elbows just above shoulder level

5. Return to the start position

MODIFIED
Use a lighter hand weight
When lifting your arms to the side, don't lift as high

ADVANCED
Use a heavier hand weight

1. Stand with your feet together and your hands down by your side

2. In one motion, jump your feet out to the side and raise your arms to the side, clapping your hands over your head

3. Immediately reverse the movement, jumping your feet back together and bringing your arms back down by your side

MODIFIED
Step your feet to the side as your arms are raised, alternating your feet each time

ADVANCED
Move faster
Add ankle and/or wrist weights

TOE TAPS

1. Start In a push-up position

2. Hold your tummy in tight

3. Alternating opposite arms and legs, bring your left knee in to your chest and tap your toe with your right hand

4. Return to starting position

5. Bring your right knee in to your chest and tap your toe with your left hand

6. Return to starting position

MODIFIED
If you can't move once in push-up position, concentrate on building your strength in this position before moving on.
As you get stronger, alternate opposite hands and feet and tap the floor, taking your hand closer to your foot each time you try. You will get there

ADVANCED
Add ankle and/or wrist weights

OVERHEAD HIGH KNEES

1. From a standing position, hold your arms straight up above your head

2. Start running on the spot, bringing your knees level with your hips

MODIFIED
March on the spot with your arms straight up over your head

ADVANCED
Hold a straight bar over your head. A broom or mop will work for this

SCISSORS

1. Lay on the floor with your hands placed on the side of your head (never behind your head)

2. Keeping your legs straight, raise your feet off the floor

3. Bring your head and shoulders off the floor

4. Bend your right leg, twisting to bring your left elbow to meet the right knee

5. Straighten this leg as you bend your left leg up at the same time as twisting your body to bring your right elbow across to meet the knee

6. Continue for the stated time

MODIFIED
Keep the straight leg on the floor as you bring the other knee up
Reduce the range of motion, taking your elbow as close to your knee as you can if you can't touch the two together

ADVANCED
Concentrate on the squeeze at the top of the move as your elbow and knee meet
Swap between a fast and slow movement, fast for 5 seconds, slow for 10 seconds for the stated time
Add ankle and/or wrist weights

STANDING OBLIQUE CRUNCH

1. Standing with feet wider than shoulder width apart

2. Place your left hand on your hip

3. Raise your right arm to the side above your head

4. Lower your right elbow down at the same time as bending your leg and bringing your right knee up to meet your elbow

5. Repeat on right for the stated time before repeating on the left

MODDIFIED
Reduce your range of motion, taking your elbow and knee as close together as you can
Hold onto a chair or wall for balance

ADVANCED
Add ankle and/or wrist weights

HIGH KNEE ANKLE TAPS

1. From a standing position, run on the spot, taking your knees up level with your hips

2. As each leg come up, tap the ankle with the opposite hand

MODIFIED
March on the spot, tapping as far down your leg as you can each time you try

ADVANCED
Move faster

HAND TO TOE TAPS

1. Lay on the floor with straight legs, arms on the floor over your head
2. Raise your head and shoulders off the floor
3. Raise your right leg and right arm about 1 inch off the floor
4. Keeping both straight, raise the right arm and leg, tapping your leg
5. Immediately return right arm and leg, keeping them both off the floor
6. Immediately repeat for the stated time before repeating on the left

MODIFIED
Keep You head and shoulders on the floor
Return your leg to the floor each time

ADVANCED
Add ankle and/or wrist weights

RUSSIAN TWISTS

1. Sit on the floor with your legs bent in front of you, feet flat on the floor
2. Place your hands under your knees and lean back until your arms are straight (you should feel the tension in your stomach in this position)
3. Take your hands from under your knees and pick up a hand weight
4. Lift your feet off the floor
5. Twist side to side, taking the weight to the left and right for thee stated time

MODIFIED
Use a lighter weight
Leave your feet on the floor

ADVANCED
Use a heavier weight
Lean further back

RAINBOW LIFTS

1. Stand with feet wider than shoulder width apart

2. Hold a hand weight in both hands in front of you, with straight arms

3. Holding your tummy in tight, lower the weight to your left foot

4. Maintaining a straight arm, raise your body and lift your straight arms diagonally over head to the right

5. Maintaining a straight arm, lower your body and straight arms, taking the weight back down to your left foot

6. Repeat for the stated time before repeating on the other side

MODIFIED
Use a lighter weight
Reduce the range of motion, taking the weight as low down as you can each time you try

ADVANCED
Use a heavier weight

HALF TO FULL SQUAT

1. Standing with your feet shoulder width apart, feet facing forward

2. Lower your body into a squat

3. Pushing through the heels of your feet, raise your body half way up

4. Immediately lower your body back to a squat

5. Pushing through the heels of your feet, immediately raise your body to starting position, squeezing your glutes at the top

6. Repeat from beginning

MODIFIED
Reduce the range of motion, taking yourself as low into your squat as you can, trying to get lower each time you try
Hold onto a chair or wall for support

ADVANCE
Add a weight, holding a weight in each hand either at your side or on your shoulders

SIDE LUNGE TO ANKLE TAP

1. Stand with feet together, tummy held tight

2. Step your right leg out to the side, lowering your body into a side lunge

3. Pushing off your right foot, pull your body back to a standing position

4. Bend your right leg up to tap your ankle with your left hand

5. From this position, return your right leg straight back out to the side, immediately lowering your body back into the side lunge

6. Repeat on right leg for the stated time before repeating on left leg

MODIFIED
Reduce the range of motion, taking yourself as low as you can in the side lunge each time you try
Remove the ankle tap, instead coming back to a standing position, balancing yourself by tapping your toes lightly on the floor before returning to the side lunge

ADVANCED
Add ankle and/or wrist weights
Add a resistance band around your ankles

SUPERMAN LEG FLUTTERS

1. Lay on the floor on your tummy with your legs straight

2. Bend your arms in front of you to rest your forehead on

3. With a flexed foot, lift your feet about one inch off the floor

4. Moving from your glutes, flutter your legs up and down, raising as much as your leg off the floor as you can

MODIFIED
Keep the flutter movement small

ADVANCED
Add ankle weights
Add a resistance band around your ankles

FRONT LUNGE TO REAR LUNGE

1. Standing with your feet together tummy pulled in tight

2. Step your right foot forward, placing your foot on the floor, lower your body to a front lunge

3. Pushing off your right foot, bring your right leg back, taking it directly behind you and lowering yourself into a rear lunge

4. Pushing off your toes, bring your right leg forward, taking it immediately into a front lunge

5. Without touching the floor, continue for the stated time before repeating with your left leg

MODIFIED
Use a chair or wall for balance
Allow your foot to tap the floor between front and rear lunges for balance

ADVANCED
Hold a hand weight in each hand
Add ankle weights

SQUAT TO FRONT KICK

1. Standing with your feet shoulder width apart and arms bent in front of you

2. Lower your body into a squat

3. As you return to a standing position, lift your left leg, kicking it out in front of you

4. Return your left foot to the floor

5. Immediately, lower your body into a squat

6. As you return to a standing position, lift your right leg, kicking it out in front of you

7. Continue to alternate legs for stated time

MODIFIED
Keep your squats higher and your kicks lower
Hold onto a chair or wall for balance

ADVANCED
Add ankle and/or wrist weights

SQUAT TO FRONT LUNGE

1. Standing with your feet shoulder width apart
2. Lower your body into a squat
3. As you return to a standing position, step your right foot forward
4. Immediately lower your body to a front lunge
5. Pushing off your right foot comeback to standing position, placing your right foot back to the floor
6. Immediately lower your body into a squat
7. Continue on your right leg for stated time before repeating on your left leg

MODIFIED
Don't move as fast
Reduce your range of motion, getting lower in your squats and lunges each time you try

ADVANCED
Move faster
Jump from squat to lunge and from lunge to squat
Add ankle weights

BENT OVER LEG EXTENSION

1. Stand facing a chair
2. Bend over with a slight bend in your knees, holding the back of the chair for support
3. With a flexed foot, moving from your glutes, raise your right leg until level with your back
4. Return your leg to starting position
5. Continue move on right leg for stated time before repeating with your left leg

MODIFIED
Don't bend over as far
Don't raise your leg as high

ADVANCED
Add ankle weights
Add a resistance band around your ankles

PLIE POWER SQUAT

1. Standing with feet together, tummy held in tight

2. Jump your feet out to the side, landing in a plie squat with toes facing outward and at the same time, as you land, take your left hand down to your right foot

3. Jump back to standing position with your feet together

4. Jump your feet out to the side, landing in a plie squat with toes facing outward and at the same time as you land, this time take your right hand down to your right foot

5. Jump back to standing position with your feet together

6. Continue for stated time, alternating feet to hands

MODIFIED
Remove the jump, lowering your body into a plie squat, taking your hands as close to your feet as you can

ADVANCED
Move faster
Add ankle and/or wrist weights

PLIE HALF TO FULL SQUAT

1. Standing With feet wider than shoulder width apart, toes pointing outward

2. Lower your body into a plie squat, keeping your chest and shoulders up

3. Raise your body half way to standing position

4. Immediately lower your body back into a plie squat

5. Raise your body to starting position

6. Immediately lower back into plie

7. Continue with half raise then full raise for the stated time

MODIFIED
Reduce your range of motion, lowering as far you can each time you try
Hold onto a chair or wall for balance

ADVANCED
Add a hand weight in each hand, holding either in front of you or on your shoulders

PLANK HIP TWISTS

1. Starting in plank position, hold your tummy in tight

2. Twist your hip s to the right, lowering them to the floor

3. Twist your hips straight over to the left, lowering them to the floor

4. Continue, twisting your hips to the left and right for the stated time

MODIFIED
Reduce the range of motion, lowering your hips as far as you can each time you try
Break the time down, trying to complete smaller chunks of time until you can build up to the stated duration

ADVANCED
Move faster, getting as many twists in as you can during the stated time

SQUAT TO FRONT ARM RAISE

1. Holding a hand weight in each hand, held in front of your body

2. Stand with feet shoulder width apart

3. Lower your body into a squat

4. As you return to starting position, with a straight arm, raise both arms at the same time in front of you, level with your shoulders

5. Lower your arms and immediately lower your body into a squat

6. Continue for stated time

MODIFIED
Use a lighter weight
Reduce the range of motion squatting lower each time you try

ADVANCED
Use a heavier weight

WIDE IN/OUT ABS

1. Starting in a push-up position
2. Take your feet wide
3. Jump your feet in towards your hands
4. Immediately jump your feet back to starting position
5. Continue for stated time

MODIFIED
From starting position, step your feet in and out

ADVANCED
Move faster
Bring your feet closer to your hands
Add ankle weights

PLIE SQUAT SPEED JABS

1. Standing with your feet wider than shoulder width apart, toes pointing outward
2. Lower your body into a plie squat
3. Raise your arms up with a clenched fist
4. Alternate left and right punches as fast as you can, maintaining the plie squat throughout

MODIFIED
Don't take your plie squat as low
Slow down

ADVANCED
Hold a hand weight in each hand
Add wrist weights
Move faster

1. Standing with feet together, hands up in front of you
2. Jump your feet out to the side into a plie squat, toes pointing outward
3. At the same time, swing your right arm to the side into a hook punch
4. Immediately jump your feet back to starting position, returning your arm to starting position
5. Immediately jump your feet out to the side into a plie squat, toes pointing outward
6. At the same time, swing your left arm to the side into a hook punch
7. Immediately jump your feet back to the starting position, returning your arm to the starting position
8. Continue, alternating hook punches for the stated time

MODIFIED
Remove the jump, lowering your body into plie squat as you hook punch

ADVANCED
Move faster
Add a hand weight into each hand
Add wrist weights

1. Standing with feet together, hands down by your side
2. Jump your feet forward and backward in a scissor movement (as your left foot goes forward, your right foot goes back)
3. At the same time, raise your arms up and down in a scissors movement (as your left arm goes up and forward, your right arm goes down)

MODIFIED
Remove the jumping, step your left foot forward and raise your right arm
Swap over, stepping your right foot forward and raising your left arm

ADVANCED
Move faster
Add ankle and/or wrist weights

SQUAT TO REAR KICK

1. Standing with your feet shoulder width apart and arms bent in front of you, elbows raised to the front

2. Lower your body into a squat

3. As you return to a standing position, lift your left leg, kicking it out behind you

4. Return your left foot to the floor

5. Immediately, lower your body into a squat

6. As you return to a standing position, left your right leg, kicking it out behind you

7. Continue to alternate legs for stated time

MODIFIED
Keep your squats higher
Keep your kicks lower
Hold onto a chair or wall for balance

ADVANCED
Move faster
Add ankle and/or wrist weights

8 CORE COUNT

1. In a standing position repeat the following moves for a count of 8 on each

2. High knees (running on spot bringing knees level with hips)

3. Sprinting (running on spot as fast as you can)

4. Floor Sprints (drop to the floor and floor sprint as fast as you can)

5. Jump back to starting position as fast as you can and repeat without rest

6. Continue for stated time

MODIFIED
Remove the floor sprints and reduce the speed of the remaining moves, completing each one for count of 8: March on spot, bringing knees up level with hips. Run on spot.

ADVANCED
Move as fast as you can, moving from one position to the next quickly
Add ankle and/or wrist weights

SUPERMAN LEG TAPS

1. Lay on the floor on your tummy with your legs straight and arms down by your side

2. Raise your chest off the floor

3. Bend down your left side, tapping your leg as low down the leg as you can

4. Bend straight over down your right side, tapping your leg as far down your leg as you can

5. Continue bending left and right, tapping as low down each leg as you can for the stated time

MODIFIED
Keep the movement slower
Tap higher up the leg

ADVANCED
Move faster
Tap further down the leg

KERI'S WORDS

When I was pregnant with my third baby, my body changed completely and I thought I would never get my pre-children body back. Well, after following this programme I did just that. Because the programme showed me how to train effectively at home and gave me the recipes to cook family meals that everyone at home would eat, which meant I wasn't cooking myself one thing and my children something else. I could use this programme within my normal daily life. I didn't have to plan and prepare a whole new, different eating programme. I think it was because of this that made this programme so easy to implement into my existing routine and sustainable within our family life. This programme proved fantastic for us all because not only did I achieve my own body and weight loss goals, but my children benefited too because I was serving them the same healthy meals that I was eating too. The L.I.F.E. Fit programme is more than just a weight loss programme. I can't tell you the difference it has made to our family. I have had a crazy busy year with lots of friends getting married and thanks to this programme, I have been able to enjoy the hen parties in the sun feeling great and confident running around in my bikini with my fellow hens. I am so happy"

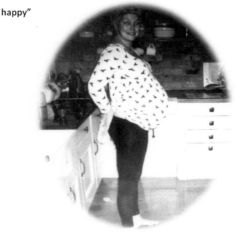
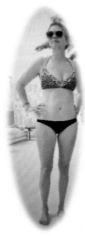

"I have never been overweight but after having my second baby, I wanted to lose my baby weight and tone my body again. Since following the L.I.F.E. Fit programme, I have never felt better. My body is more toned and lifted now than it has ever been. I have always done various gym group classes and boot camps but this is the most toned and defined my body has ever been. Even my husband notices the difference. I love how the exercises adapt to my fitness level so just when I am easing through a routine, they are changed to challenge me again, designed to constantly improve my fitness level and body tone. The programme has taught me a healthy way of life, without living in the gym. My whole family are benefiting from it, without having to follow a strict food regime. I can cook the same meal for the whole family, which makes life easier with two young children and the best thing is, my children are growing up seeing me enjoying a healthy, active and balanced lifestyle. I love it and I love the lifestyle this programme creates"

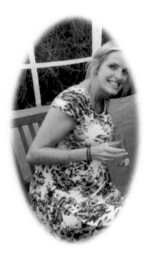 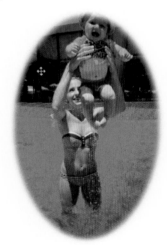

You should consult your doctor or other health care professional before starting this or any other fitness programme to determine if it is right for your needs. This is particularly true if you (or your family) have a history of high blood pressure or heart disease, or if you have ever experienced chest pain when exercising or have experienced chest pain in the past month when not engaged in physical activity or if you smoke, have high cholesterol, are obese or have a bone or joint problem that could be made worse by a change in physical activity. Do not start this fitness programme if your doctor or health care provider advises against it. If you experience faintness, dizziness, pain or shortness of breath at any time while exercising you should stop immediately. You should understand that when participating in any exercise or exercise programme, there is the possibility of physical injury. If you engage in this fitness programme, you agree that you do so at your own risk, are voluntarily participating in these activities and assume all risk of injury to yourself.

Printed in Germany
by Amazon Distribution
GmbH, Leipzig